MW01614617

CONSUMER'S GUIDE TO CHILDHOOD VACCINES

Barbara Loe Fisher
National Vaccine Information Center

Published by:
The National Vaccine Information Center

Requests for permission should be mailed to:
    Permissions, National Vaccine Information Center
    512 W. Maple Ave., Suite 206, Vienna, Virginia 22180.

Library of Congress Catalog Card Number
ISBN 1-889204-01-3

Editor: Barbara Loe Fisher
Associate Editor: Kathi Williams

Printed in the United States of America

TABLE OF CONTENTS

NOTE TO READERS

The information in this book is for educational purposes only. It is not intended to be medical or legal advice. Those seeking medical or legal advice should obtain the services of a competent attorney, physician or qualified health care professional. The National Vaccine Information Center encourages all readers of this guide to gather additional information on diseases and vaccines and consult one or more health care professionals before making a vaccination decision.

The Front Cover Photo:
David John was a healthy four month old baby when, within hours of his second DPT shot, he displayed neurological signs and soon after developed a seizure disorder. He died in his sleep when he was two years old.

Dear Parents:

As mothers of children, who were left injured after serious reactions to the DPT vaccine, we know how important it is to be fully informed about childhood diseases and vaccines. We vaccinated our children because we wanted to protect them from the risk of becoming seriously ill from childhood diseases. We were never told there was a risk of our children becoming seriously ill from a vaccine reaction. We learned too late that our children were at high risk for reacting to the DPT vaccine and, if we had been more informed, we could have prevented our children from becoming a vaccine reaction statistic.

As co-founders of the National Vaccine Information Center, we have worked since 1982 to prevent vaccine injuries and deaths through public education. We support informed health care choices for all consumers. The National Vaccine Information Center maintains that only the least toxic and most technologically advanced vaccines should be made available to the public. At the same time, we maintain that all health care consumers should have the right to informed consent to vaccination, including the right to choose which vaccines they and their children will use.

Making informed vaccination decisions and taking responsibility for them is not easy. Sometimes it seems a lot easier to just not ask questions or simply do what someone else tells us to do. But remaining ignorant and trusting blindly can be the biggest risk of all.

Whatever decision you make, you are being the very best mother or father that you can be by taking the time to learn more. There is no greater gift we can give to our children than to be willing to ask the hard questions and make the hard choices that will affect the rest of their lives until they are old enough to ask those questions and make those choices for themselves.

With kindest regards,

Barbara Loe Fisher, Co-Founder & President
Kathi Williams, Co-Founder & Director

INTRODUCTION

The following information has been developed by the National Vaccine Information Center (NVIC), a non-profit organization founded in 1982 and dedicated to preventing vaccine injuries and deaths through public education. The oldest and largest national organization advocating the right for citizens to make informed vaccination decisions, the National Vaccine Information Center represents health care consumers and health care professionals as well as individuals who have been affected by vaccine reactions, injuries and deaths, including parents of vaccine injured children. NVIC supports the right of consumers to have access to the least toxic and most technologically advanced vaccines as well as the right to make informed, independent vaccination decisions for themselves and their children.

MAKE AN EDUCATED VACCINATION DECISION

This information is not intended to substitute for medical advice provided to you by your physician. It will not tell you to vaccinate or not to vaccinate. This information will help you become better educated about diseases and vaccines in order to help you make a more informed vaccination decision.

It is important to be equally concerned and knowledgeable about diseases and vaccines. Your challenge as a health care consumer is to determine what is the best course of action to take based on personal medical history, family medical history, current health status, disease severity and incidence rates, vaccine reaction data, and your personal beliefs. You should make this decision after consulting with your doctor, who is required by law to provide you with information, after considering your state's vaccination laws and after reviewing information from other sources, including additional information our organization can provide to you.

Chapter One

UNIVERSALLY REQUIRED CHILDHOOD VACCINES

Government recommended vaccines mandated by most states in the U.S. include:

DPT or DTaP: Diphtheria, pertussis (also known as whooping cough) and tetanus inactivated bacterial vaccines combined into the DPT or DTaP shot. DTaP vaccine, licensed for infants in 1996, contains a purified pertussis vaccine with fewer toxins in it.

MMR: Measles, mumps and rubella live viral vaccines combined into the MMR shot.

Polio: Usually given in live oral vaccine form known as OPV. An inactivated poliovirus vaccine known as IPV is also available in injectable form. In 1996 the government changed its polio vaccine policy to recommend that the first two doses of polio vaccine be IPV and the second two doses be OPV. However, an all-IPV or all-OPV schedule is also accepted.

In addition to DPT, MMR and Polio vaccines, many states also require children to have:

HIB: Haemophilus influenza type b bacterial vaccine in order to attend day care or kindergarten. (A Hib vaccine combined with DPT vaccine into one shot called DPTH is routinely being given to infants and children under five. There is also a combination Hib and hepatitis B vaccine licensed in 1996 that is being offered to infants and children).

HEP-B: Hepatitis B inactivated virus vaccine is routinely given in hospital newborn nurseries before babies are discharged to go home. By 1996, 19 states had laws requiring its use by children and teenagers.

Varicella Zoster: (chicken pox) live virus vaccine, licensed in 1995, is not yet mandated by most states but the government recommends all individuals over one year, who have not had chicken pox, get it.

In addition, the government recommends some children and adults get inactivated **hepatitis A** virus vaccine, **pneumococcal** (pneumonia) bacterial vaccine, and inactivated **influenza** (flu) virus vaccine.

Chapter Two

RECOMMENDED VACCINATION SCHEDULES

Recommended vaccination schedules are developed by the federal government through the Centers for Disease Control (CDC) in the Department of Health and Human Services and by the American Academy of Pediatrics (AAP), a medical organization representing private pediatricians. Most state legislatures follow CDC or AAP guidelines in their mandatory vaccination laws. The customary schedule for giving childhood vaccines is:

DPT or DTaP vaccine at 2, 4, 6, 18 months old and a booster between 4 and 6 years old. Not recommended after the seventh birthday.

DT or Td vaccine. DT vaccine is given at 2, 4, 6, and 18 months old to children who cannot receive the pertussis portion of DPT or DTaP vaccine. DT vaccine is given up to the seventh birthday. A Td booster shot is recommended at 11-12 years if it has been at least 5 years since the last DPT, DTaP or DT shots.

Polio vaccine: **IPV** at 2 and 4 months; **OPV** vaccine at 6 months old and booster between 4 and 6 years old. An all -OPV or all -IPV schedule is also accepted.

MMR vaccine at 15 months old. Many states also require a **measles** booster shot either before entry to kindergarten or before entry to junior high school.

HIB vaccine at 2, 4, 6 and 12-15 months old. Recommendations state Hib shots should be given at least 2 months apart. Not every state requires this vaccine and most do not require it after 36 months of age. If the first Hib vaccination is given after 15 months, only one dose is recommended. Not recommended after fifth birthday.

Hep B vaccine at birth with follow-up boosters at 1 and 6 months. Recommendations state that doses one and two should be at least 1 month apart and the third dose should be given at least 4 months after the first dose.

Varicella Zoster vaccine given in one dose at 12 to 18 months of age. For children over 13 years who have not been vaccinated and have never had chicken pox, two doses 1 to 2 months apart are recommended.

Chapter Three

DISEASES:
THEIR SYMPTOMS AND COMPLICATIONS

As an informed health care consumer, you have an equal responsibility to become educated about the infectious diseases which vaccines are designed to prevent. Whooping cough, tetanus, haemophilus influenzae type b and other diseases can, in an individual case, injure or kill depending upon the disease, the individual's general health, nutritional and environmental status, genetic predisposition and medical treatment options.

Mass vaccination during the past 40-years has altered the natural epidemiology of many childhood diseases and some, like measles and mumps, are now more frequently occurring in older teenagers and adults when they can be more serious. It is important to know the symptoms of these diseases and their complications.

At the end of this book, there is a GLOSSARY OF MEDICAL TERMS that describes health problems associated with diseases and vaccination, The GLOSSARY will help you identify a vaccine reaction or a health problem which may be related to vaccination or disease complications.

DIPHTHERIA: In the 18th and early 19th centuries, diphtheria was a widespread and feared disease but was on a decline at the turn of this century. In 1921, 206,939 cases were reported in the U.S., the highest number ever reported in one year. In 1992, there were only 4 cases reported in the U.S. with 1 death.

Diphtheria is caused by a bacterium found in the mouth, throat and nose of the infected person. It is spread by coughing and sneezing. Persons who appear healthy can be "carriers" of the disease. Diphtheria occurs most frequently in the winter and, while rare during the first six months of life, tends to be more common in children between the ages of two and five years old.

Diphtheria is usually treated with the use of diphtheria antitoxin, antibiotics, oxygen and tracheotomy to open the windpipe. However, if treatment is inadequate or does not begin in time, a powerful toxin produced by the diphtheria bacteria may spread throughout the body. In underdeveloped countries with poor nutrition, sanitation and healthcare, diphthe-

Symptoms of diphtheria are similar to croup, with noisy breathing, hoarseness and cough, sore throat, slight fever, chills and irritability with increasing inability to breathe caused by a grayish membrane that covers the tonsils and throat. If the membrane continues to grow, it can interfere with swallowing. If it extends to the windpipe, it can block the passage of air and cause suffocation.

ria can be very serious. Diphtheria can lead to circulatory complications with heart and kidney damage and broncho-pneumonia. Paralysis of eye muscles, palate and other parts of the body as well as heart failure and death can also occur.

PERTUSSIS (WHOOPING COUGH): Pertussis, or whooping cough, as it is commonly known, is often called the "100 day cough" and is highly contagious. At the turn of this century, whooping cough had become less deadly and was on the decline in technologically advanced countries even though it was still widespread and most American children experienced a bout before the age of ten. Depending upon the general health of the person as well as other unknown factors, a bout with whooping cough in the U.S. today can be mild or severe. Recovery from whooping cough often confers permanent immunity, although sometimes people who have had whooping cough may have a milder case again.

In 1934, there were 265,269 cases of pertussis reported in the U.S., the highest number of cases reported in one year. During the last several years, there have been between 3,000 and 7,000 cases of pertussis reported annually in the U.S., but it is thought that these figures only represent 10 to 20 percent of actual cases. In 1992, there were 4,083 pertussis cases reported in the U.S. with 5 deaths. A cyclical disease with natural increases every three to four years in countries around the world no matter how high the vaccination rate in the population, whooping cough is most dangerous in Third World countries or in underprivileged communities in technologically advanced countries with poor living conditions, sanitation, nutrition and substandard health care. There are other respiratory diseases caused by different bacteria and viruses that can mimic whooping cough so lab test confirmation is important to make a definitive diagnosis.

Pertussis is caused by a bacterium found in the mouth, nose and throat of an infected person and is spread through coughing and sneezing. Vaccinated persons can get whooping cough because vaccine acquired immunity wears off in older children and adults; however in older children or adults symptoms are often milder, such as an irritating cough that won't go away or a more severe cough (coughing so hard the stomach muscles and ribs hurt) without the characteristic 'whoop." These unsuspecting infected older children and adults, who are often misdiagnosed as having bronchitis, a bad cold or the flu, can then pass the disease along to the more vulnerable younger children and babies.

Whooping cough is most dangerous for younger children because it causes severe paroxysmal spells of coughing which can interfere with eating, drinking and breathing. The younger the child and the smaller the air passages, the more dangerous the disease. Several toxins produced by the pertussis bacteria are responsible for producing the thick, sticky mucus that can clog the tiny airways of small children and block the passage of air, causing them to cough violently and then make a "whoop" sound as they gasp and try to take in air through their clogged airways.

Following an incubation period of 6 to 20 days, a typical progression of the disease in young children starts with a short, dry persistent cough that may appear to be nothing more than a slight cold. Often there is no runny nose, sore throat or fever, which may cause the parent to think the cough is an allergy. Cough syrup and other over-the-counter medicines will not stop the cough from progressing. The cough persists and starts to worsen at about day ten or twelve as mucus production begins to increase. At this point, the child may begin to run a slight fever (99.5 F.) and may refuse to eat or drink very much and will begin to cough more at night.

Children with whooping cough may appear to be fine during the day and play normally between bouts of coughing. However, eating, drinking and any physical activity such as running can cause prolonged coughing

By the end of the second week and into the third week, the child with whooping cough may begin to cough violently, especially at night between the hours of 11 p.m. and 5 a.m., and will appear to be "drowning" in mucus that will be vomited up through the mouth and nose at the end of coughing spells. The child may be unable to keep down liquids or solid foods. The vomiting and running of a persistent low grade fever that cannot be brought down by the use of fever reducing medicines, can cause the child to lose weight, become dehydrated and weak. Children are often encouraged to drink liquids during the day between coughing spells and to take naps to make up for sleep lost during the night.

spells, gagging and vomiting. During weeks three and four when the disease is most severe, there may be times at night when the child awakens choking and, trying to dislodge the mucus, the eyes will bulge and the face will turn blue from lack of oxygen before the child is able to take in a breath. Many parents have reported sleeping near their children to care for them during the weeks when the disease is most severe.

Frequently, the antibiotic, erythromycin, is prescribed for those infected with pertussis. This antibiotic is thought to be most useful in reducing the spread of the disease and in preventing secondary infections such as pneumonia. There is some evidence that if erythromycin is given either before any coughing begins or shortly after slight coughing begins (week one), that it may eliminate infection, prevent disease and reduce spread of the disease to others. However, in most cases, antibiotics and over-the-counter cough and cold medicines cannot alter the course of the disease, especially after paroxysmal coughing has begun.

Some parents have reported success in modifying whooping cough symptoms through the use of homeopathic and naturopathic remedies. Traditional Chinese Medicine (including acupuncture) has also been used. Chiropractic adjustment or osteopathic manipulation has reportedly helped to facilitate breathing. Parents report that the sooner these remedies and adjustments are begun, the better the chance for modifying the symptoms and helping to speed recovery.

Small babies with severe cases of whooping cough are often hospitalized and given respiratory assistance, including suctioning of mucus from the throat in order to resuscitate them after they stop breathing between coughing spells. Intravenous rehydration therapy is also used to replace lost body fluids. In some children and adults, nosebleeds, hemorrhage in the eyes, bruised ribs and sore muscles can occur from prolonged, forceful coughing. Occasionally, convulsions, inflammation of the brain and death can occur. Secondary infections such as pneumonia, bronchitis and otitis media are more common and can be quite severe if left untreated. Bacterial pneumonia kills most children under the age of three who receive inadequate treatment or live in substandard living conditions.

Whooping cough, together with its secondary respiratory complications, can last from two to four months with the most serious coughing lasting two to three weeks. Because whooping cough is highly contagious, especially during the first few weeks, infected individuals should be isolated from others as soon as the disease is suspected or confirmed through a lab culture or blood test. Most children are able to be treated at home but others, especially those under age five, may have to be hospitalized during the most severe course of the disease.

TETANUS: Tetanus, commonly called lockjaw, is caused by a bacterium that is mostly present in soil, manure, and in the digestive tracts of humans and animals. Tetanus bacteria enter the body through a wound - sometimes as small as a pinprick or deep scratch but most often through a deep puncture wound or laceration such as those made by rusty nails or dirty knives. Such wounds are difficult to clean adequately and, if teta-

The incubation period for symptoms of tetanus to begin can range from one to three weeks. The first symptoms are likely to be headache, irritability, fever, chills, and muscular stiffness of the jaw and neck. As the poison increases and spreads, the body becomes rigid and locked in spasm with head drawn back, legs and feet extended, arms stiff, hands clenched and the jaw unable to open with difficulty in swallowing. The stomach muscles also become rigid and convulsions may occur.

nus bacteria were present on the nail or knife, the bacteria can remain deep in the wound where they can grow and produce several toxins that attack the body's red and white blood cells and central nervous system. Tetanus bacteria do not grow well in the presence of oxygen, which is why deep puncture wounds are a perfect environment for them to grow.

Immediate hospitalization and the use of tetanus antitoxin and powerful tranquilizers and anti-spasmodic drugs are used to treat the disease. The symptoms last for several weeks. Complications of tetanus include pneumonia, bone fractures from violent muscle spasms and death.

In 1948, there were 601 cases of tetanus reported in the U.S., the highest number of cases reported in one year. In 1992, there were 45 cases of tetanus and 9 deaths reported in the U.S.. Tetanus is a much more serious problem in underdeveloped countries, especially among newborn babies born in unsanitary conditions whose umbilical cords can become infected with tetanus.

POLIO: Polio emerged as a significant disease during the latter part of the nineteenth century and caused widespread panic in the U.S. in the 1950's. In 1952, there were 21,269 cases of wild polio reported in the U.S., the highest number of cases reported in one year. Polio continues to be present in Third World countries, although it is reported to be eradicated in the western hemisphere. Since 1979, the only cases of polio reported to be occurring in the U.S. today are caused by the live oral polio vaccine, which health officials have given credit for eliminating the wild poliovirus in the U.S.

Poliomyelitis is caused by several different types of polioviruses that live in the nose, throat and, especially, the intestinal tract of a person infected with it. The incubation period is usually between one and two weeks. The wild poliovirus produces varying symptoms and degrees of neurological signs and complications, depending upon the type of polio virus involved. According to infectious disease experts, approximately one percent of wild polio infections results in paralytic disease.

Most wild virus infections are mild and the milder forms of polio usually begin abruptly and last, at most, a few days. When symptoms are present, they include fever, sore throat, nausea, headache and stomach ache. Sometimes the individual will feel pain and stiffness in the neck,

14

back and legs. Usually there is full recovery with no muscular or nerve damage. The vast majority of children and adults who got polio in the 1950's recovered from this milder type of polio.

In spinal poliomyelitis, there is weakness and pain of the neck, abdomen, diaphragm and arms and legs because the virus affects the surrounding nerves. Initial symptoms can include minor upper respiratory infection, fever, headache, sore throat, vomiting, diarrhea, stiff neck and pain when extending the legs or moving the head. The symptoms can disappear gradually and no permanent damage occurs.

In bulbar polio, one or more cranial nerves and the centers of respiration and circulation are involved. Symptoms include difficulty swallowing and breathing. When trying to drink fluids, inability to swallow will cause the fluids to flow out of the nose. Paralysis of the respiratory system makes it necessary for the individual to be placed on a respirator and often a tracheotomy is performed to open up the windpipe.

Encephalitic polio symptoms include disorientation, drowsiness, irritability and tremors. A spinal tap is used to diagnose this type of polio.

In the more severe forms of wild polio, paralysis, which usually occurs within the first week, can become permanent and occasionally end in death. There is no specific treatment for polio other than physical therapy. Recovery rates vary. Some individuals recover with mild disabilities or none at all. Others may be permanently paralyzed or die.

In children under five years old, wild polio most commonly can cause weakness or paralysis in one leg. In children ages 5 to 15, weakness of one arm or one arm and leg is likely. In adults, paralysis of both legs and arms and bladder and respiratory damage is also frequent. Severe pain in the affected areas is also a common long term effect. Some people, who recovered from polio in the 1950's are now suffering from "post-polio syndrome," a condition that includes extreme chronic fatigue, muscle weakness and other neurological signs.

Because the oral polio vaccine (OPV) given to most children is a live virus vaccine (the IPV or inactivated, injectable polio vaccine cannot transmit polio), it can give vaccine strain polio to the child who receives it,

15

especially if the child is immune compromised. The live vaccine strain poliovirus lives in the intestinal tract of a recently vaccinated child for four to six weeks and, therefore, mothers and fathers, babysitters, playmates and other individuals who come into close contact with the child are exposed to the virus and are "passively revaccinated" without their knowledge. If the person who comes into contact with a child recently vaccinated with live polio vaccine is not immune to polio or has a suppressed immune system (for example, from chemotherapy or an immune disorder), he or she can get vaccine strain polio.

In the U.S. today, about 10 cases of vaccine associated polio are reported to occur in children and adults every year. It is thought that this is an underestimation of the actual number of cases occurring because vaccine associated polio, especially milder cases, can be misdiagnosed as other kinds of neurological dysfunction. Confirmation of vaccine associated polio can sometimes be obtained through a lab test to culture out the vaccine strain polio virus.

Unfortunately, while cases of wild polio can be mild and recovery can be complete, many of the cases of vaccine strain polio do not recover. Many children and adults, who get vaccine strain polio are quadriplegic and are on respirators. Like with severe cases of wild polio disease, death can occur from severe complications of vaccine strain polio.

MEASLES: Measles, also called rubeola, is a highly contagious disease caused by a virus and is spread by coughing, sneezing or simply breathing near another person. Measles usually is most common in the late winter and early spring. Up until the past two decades, measles was one of the most common childhood diseases in America, occurring primarily in children aged two to six years, and almost every child had measles by the age of 15.

Historically, the majority of children in technologically advanced countries recovered from measles without major complications. However, measles in teenagers and adults or in very young infants can be much more severe with serious complications and increased mortality. In 1941, there were 894,134 cases of measles reported, the highest mumber of cases ever reported in one year. In 1992 there were 2,237 cases reported in the U.S. with 4 deaths.

Some researchers believe that measles as a childhood disease in years past helped the human immune system to mature, priming it to be more effective in dealing with challenges from viruses and bacteria later in life. Recovery from natural measles infection confers lifelong immunity while vaccine-induced antibodies provide temporary immunity. A woman who has recovered from measles as a child passes maternal antibodies to her fetus, which often protects her newborn from measles for the first year of life. Young mothers today, who were vaccinated as children and never had measles do not have natural maternal measles antibodies to pass on to their babies and, so, most American babies born today are vulnerable to measles from the moment of birth.

Measles is a cyclical disease and there are increases around the world every two to three years. Measles is dangerous in Third World countries or in underprivileged communities in technologically advanced countries with poor living conditions, sanitation, nutrition and substandard health care.

The incubation period for measles is usually 10 to 20 days and the course of the disease lasts several weeks. Most cases of measles are mild and symptoms begin with a light, hacking cough, low fever, runny eyes and nose and general signs of a cold. For four or five days before the outbreak of measles spots, the cough can become more severe and hacking with swelling and redness of the eyes and sensitivity to light. Fevers can be high (104-105 F.). The symptoms of high fever and cold do not respond to antibiotics, aspirin or cough medicine.

The symptoms worsen before the rash appears and 24-49 hours before the rash appears, the inside of the mouth is covered with grayish-white dots surrounded by reddening that are about the size of a grain of salt. The rash is faint at the beginning and first appears behind the ears and then becomes darker and spreads rapidly to the face, neck and arms within 24 hours. By the time the rash reaches the legs and feet - in two to three days - it begins to fade on the face and gradually fades from the rest of the body in the next few days. As soon as the rash appears, the child appears to be much better.

Treatment includes soothing applications to relieve the itchy rash and fluids, cool sponge baths and other therapy to help reduce fever and prevent dehydration. Other health care therapies, including homeopathy, naturopathy, Traditional Chinese Medicine, and chiropractic, have been used to modify the symptoms of measles and enhance the natural ability of the immune system to heal the body. Recovery from measles in a previously healthy child is usually complete without complications.

However, a severe case of measles can include secondary infections such as otitis media (inner ear infections), strep, bronchitis, pneumonia, hepatitis and Haemophilus influenza. Occasionally, extremely high fevers, brain inflammation and convulsions can be followed by permanent brain damage, transverse myelitis, subacute sclerosing panencephalitis, deafness, blindness, paralysis, and death. Complications are more common in adults, in immune compromised or chronically ill children and in babies under one year old.

An atypical, severe form of measles has been seen in some persons who have been vaccinated with inactivated measles vaccine (not currently used in the U.S.). Symptoms begin with a fever, headache and stomach pain for several days and then a rash appears on the hands and feet and progresses towards the head - just the opposite progression that is seen in natural measles. The rash is especially noticeable on the legs and in body creases. Severe pneumonia is a common complication. Live virus measles vaccine, which is licensed for use in the U.S. today, can sometimes cause vaccine strain measles virus infection, which is very severe and can end in death.

MUMPS: Mumps is a viral disease that can be spread through coughing, sneezing or simply breathing near another person. It used to be a very common childhood disease in the U.S. among children under age ten. In 1968, there were 152,209 cases reported, the highest number of cases ever reported in one year. In 1994 only about 1,500 cases were reported. A usually mild disease in children, it can be much more severe in older teenagers and adults.

Mumps can cause fever, headache and inflammation of the salivary glands, which makes the cheeks swell. Incubation is generally 14 to 21 days. Symptoms may begin with low grade fever, headache, vomiting and earache. Swelling first appears in front of the ear above the jaw line but the glands under the chin can also be involved. Eating is painful because the saliva irritates swollen glands. Just one side or both sides of the face may swell. Swelling usually goes away in a week and recovery is usually complete without complications.

18

Rarely, mumps can be more severe and cause an inflammation of the lining of the brain and spinal cord (meningitis). Symptoms include severe headache, vomiting, irritability, lethargy. Rarely, it can cause inflammation of the brain itself and can cause permanent brain damage, deafness or death (one death was reported in 1991). Adolescent or adult males who get mumps can develop painful inflammation and swelling of the testicles (orchitis) and, in rare cases, become sterile.

Treatment for mumps infection includes bed rest, bland diet and plenty of fluids. Other health care therapies such as homeopathic, naturopathic, Traditional Chinese Medicine and chiropractic have been used to modify the symptoms of mumps and enhance the functioning of the immune system. Recovery from mumps infection confers lifelong immunity.

RUBELLA: Also known as German Measles or the "three day measles," rubella is usually a mild childhood disease and used to be common in American children five to nine years old. However, today in the U.S., rubella is most frequently seen among teenagers and young adults when it can be more serious.

In 1969, there were 57,686 cases of rubella reported in the U.S., the highest number of cases reported in one year. In 1992, there were 160 cases of rubella reported in the U.S. with one death reported to have resulted from disease complications. In 1994, there were 227 cases, with 171 (75 percent) occurring in adults more than 20-years old.

Rubella is a cyclical disease and increases are seen around the world every six to nine years. It occurs most often in the winter and spring and is spread through coughing, sneezing or simply breathing near another person. The virus can be found in an infected person's blood and throat.

Incubation period is 14 to 21 days. Symptoms begin with signs of a mild cold, low-grade fever and swelling of the glands in the back of the neck and under the chin. Sometimes the glands behind the ears become enlarged. A pink rash first appears on the face and then spreads to the arms, head, chest and sometimes the legs. The rash is not as red or blotchy as measles and generally fades by the third to fifth day. Recovery from rubella usually confers lifelong immunity, although repeat cases do occur rarely.

19

If a woman gets rubella in the first trimester of pregnancy, she has a 20 to 25 percent greater chance of giving birth to a deformed baby and is at risk of suffering a miscarriage. Birth defects can include blindness, damage to the heart and major arteries, deafness, abnormaly small brain and mental retardation.

Young adults, especially young women, who get rubella may have swollen glands in the back of the neck and some pain, swelling and stiffness in the joints (arthritis) that persists for several weeks. Recovery from rubella is usually quick but occasionally brain inflammation and chronic arthritis can cause permanent damage.

HAEMOPHILUS INFLUENZA TYPE B (HIB): Haemophilus influenza type b bacteria was first isolated in 1892 from victims in an influenza epidemic. This bacteria lives in the human respiratory tract and can be recovered from the nasal and throat passages of up to 90 percent of all healthy individuals. But today American children aged 6 to 48 months are highly susceptible to developing Hib infection, especially if they are immune compromised or live in crowded, substandard living conditions. Hib disease is spread through sneezing, coughing or inhaling respiratory tract secretions of an infected person. Hib infections occur most often during the late winter and spring.

Historically, Hib disease has been rare in newborns and adults, although the incidence of Hib disease increased fourfold between the years 1946 and 1986 and more adults have became vulnerable. The reason for the sudden increase in the incidence and severity of Hib disease in this century is unknown. However, some scientists believe that excessive use of antibiotics may have caused the organism to change and become more virulent. Common antibiotics, such as ampicillin, which once were used to help people recover from the disease are no longer effective treatments for Hib disease because the bacteria has become resistant to it.

Without immediate and adequate medical treatment, Hib disease has a significant death rate (5 to 10 percent) and a high rate of seizures and other neurological complications (30 percent). Other complications include pneumonia and heart involvement with long term damage including hearing loss and neurological dysfunction. Antibiotic therapy using powerful

20

antibiotics is only one part of the treatment, which may include respiratory and oxygen therapy, blood transfusions, fluid replacement, tracheostomy, and anticonvulsant therapy.

When a Hib disease case is confirmed, often both unvaccinated AND vaccinated children within the same family or classroom are given "pro-

---

Hib is the most common cause of bacterial meningitis affecting children between 6 months and 4 years of age. It is not known how long the incubation period lasts. Symptoms can begin with cough, fever, chills, lack of appetite, extreme sleepiness, vomiting and, as older children and adults can testify, a severe headache. A stiff neck or back can be a warning sign. More serious signs are mental confusion, convulsions, shock and coma. In some extremely severe cases of Hib disease, a child can die within a few hours. Some cases of otitis media, sinusitis and bronchitis are also caused by Hib organisms. A spinal tap (lumbar puncture) to examine the cerebrospinal fluid (CSF), blood and urine lab tests can confirm Hib disease.

---

phylactic" antibiotic therapy in an attempt to prevent infection. Recovery from Hib disease sometimes confers permanent immunity but sometimes it does not and the individual, especially if he or she is immune compromised, can come down with another Hib infection.

In 1984, there were 20,000 cases of Hib disease estimated to have occurred in the U.S. that year, the highest number that are thought to have occurred in one year. In 1994, there were 1,174 cases of HIB disease reported in the U.S. with 329 cases occurring in children under five years of age and 463 occurring in adults over 60 years old. In 1992, 16 deaths were reported to be due to complications from Hib infection.

HEPATITIS B - It is estimated that there are more than 200 million humans in the world infected with hepatitis B virus, a virus which affects the liver. The highest incidence of hepatitis B disease occurs in the far east and tropical countries in children under five, where up to 90 percent of the adult population has recovered from hepatitis B and 8 to 15 percent are chronically infected. Hepatitis B incidence has always been lowest in

21

the U.S. and western Europe, with only 2 to 7 percent of the population ever having been infected with the virus and less than 1 percent chronically infected. The majority of hepatitis B infections in the U.S. occur in adolescents and adults.

Hepatitis B virus is found in the body fluids of infected persons. It is spread by coming into contact with an infected person's body fluids, such as saliva, blood or semen. High risk groups include needle using drug addicts; sexually promiscuous persons (especially prostitutes and promiscuous homosexual men); health care professionals exposed to blood; prisoners and other institutionalized individuals; those who receive blood transfusions or who are on hemodialysis; and babies born to mothers infected with hepatitis B virus.

The incubation period for hepatitis B disease is thought to be from 45 to 160 days. In young children, symptoms can be mild or absent at first. Nausea, vomiting, fatigue, loss of appetite, changes in smelling and taste, rash, joint pain (arthritis), headache, and cough can precede the onset of jaundice (yellow/orange coloring of the skin) by 1 or 2 weeks. Dark urine and clay colored stools may be noticed from 1 to 5 days before the onset of jaundice. The liver can become enlarged and tender with pain in the upper right abdomen.

Most people who get hepatitis B do not have to be hospitalized and 90 percent of all patients recover completely. Treatment includes restricted physical activity, a nutritious diet and monitoring for complications. Recovery, which produces a permanent immunity to hepatitis B infection unless complications result in chronic infection, can take up to four months. The elderly, immune compromised individuals and those in general poor health or living in substandard conditions are more vulnerable to rare complications which can include severe brain inflammation, gastrointestinal bleeding, respiratory and cardiac collapse, renal and liver failure, coma and death.

Among the small percentage of persons who do not completely recover from hepatitis B disease but go on to be chronically infected, it is babies infected in the womb by their infected mothers who are at highest risk for chronic hepatitis B infection and premature death from liver disease or liver cancer. 70 to 90 percent of babies born to mothers who are infected with hepatitis B become chronically infected with the virus. U.S. babies at highest risk are those born to Alaskan natives, Pacific Islanders, and first generation immigrant mothers from Asia, Middle East, Africa, and eastern Europe.

In 1992, there were 16,126 cases of hepatitis B reported in the U.S. with 903 deaths attributed to either chronic infection or complications from an acute infection. In 1994, there were 12,517 cases reported and the Centers for Disease Control stated that "hepatitis B continues to decline in most states, primarily because of changes in high risk behaviors among injecting-drug users."

VARICELLA ZOSTER (CHICKEN POX) - Varicella zoster virus is a member of the herpesvirus family and a clinical association between varicella zoster (chicken pox) and herpes zoster (shingles) has been recognized for more than 100 years. For the majority of children, chicken pox is a mild childhood disease characterized by small round lesions on the skin. It is highly contagious and half of all cases in the U.S. occur in children between the ages of 5 and 9 with the next highest incidence in children from 1 to 4 years old. It has been estimated that only 10 percent of Americans over the age of 15 have never had chicken pox.

Chicken pox is more prevalent in the late winter and early spring. The incubation period ranges between 10 and 21 days. Children can be infectious about 48 hours before the rash begins, during the 4 to 5 days the lesions appear on the skin and until all lesions are crusted over. Symptoms begin with a rash, low-grade fever and fatigue. The lesions first appear on the chest, back and face and rapidly spread to the rest of the body. Most lesions are small and the number of lesions that appear (under 10 to many hundreds) depends upon the individual. Younger children tend to have fewer lesions compared to older children and adults.

Chicken pox skin lesions produce intense itching that can be lessened with tepid water baths, wet compresses and astringent soaks. Good hygiene with daily bathing and fingernails cut short will help reduce the chance of scratched lesions becoming infected. Homeopathic, naturopathic, Traditional Chinese Medicine and other therapies which help enhance the body's natural healing ability have also been used to reduce itching and speed recovery. It is important NOT to use aspirin to bring down a fever during chicken pox. Aspirin use during chicken pox has been associated with the development of Reye's syndrome, a sometimes fatal neurological disorder.

The great majority of American children recover from a two to three week bout with chicken pox with no complications and are left with permanent immunity to the disease. However, immune compromised children, especially those with leukemia, can have a thousand or more lesions and develop severe complications, including brain inflammation and death. When there is brain involvement, it usually occurs about 21 days after the rash appears. Encephalitis is reported in under 1 percent of children with chicken pox. Another rare complication is a severe strep infection of the skin lesions which is hard to treat with antibiotics and can be fatal. Some doctors are concerned that severe strep infections associated with chicken pox have been increasing in frequency in the past decade.

Chicken pox in teenagers and adults is a much more serious disease than it is in children. Up to 20 percent of adults who get chicken pox can develop pneumonia with a fever, chest pain, inflammation of the lungs, and persistent cough. In addition to lung and brain involvement, other complications include heart and liver problems, arthritis, and corneal lesions. Up to 30 percent of babies, born to mothers who get chicken pox within 5 days of delivery or within a few days after delivery, can die from chicken pox.

About 158,000 cases of chicken pox and 100 deaths from complications were reported in the U.S. in 1992. The Centers for Disease Control states that "approximately 3.7 million cases of varicella occur annually in the United States; of these an estimated 4 to 5 percent are reported." Although reported cases of chicken pox account for only a fraction of the total number of cases that occur every year, reports of deaths associated with chicken pox complications are estimated to be more accurate.

Your risk of contracting any disease depends on your risk of exposure to the disease.

Chapter Four

WHAT IS KNOWN AND NOT KNOWN
ABOUT VACCINATION

Vaccines theoretically work on the principle of protection by artificially stimulating the immune system to produce antibodies - small molecules of protein that attack the invading organism - to overcome a disease in the same way the natural disease stimulates immunity. Protection from disease via vaccination depends upon the theory that periodically challenging the human immune system with small amounts of inactivated (killed) viruses and bacteria or attenuated (partially inactivated) live viruses will force it to produce antibodies that will confer immunity in the same way that a bout with the natural disease confers immunity.

However, vaccines do not work in the body in the same way that natural disease works in the body. When bacteria or viruses enter the body and disease progresses in a normal way, the immune system is stimulated to produce a type of natural immunity which is often permanent. Vaccines, which are most often injected directly into the blood stream or swallowed by mouth, provide an artificial, temporary immunity. Sometimes vaccines fail to provide any immunity at all. This is why multiple doses of many viral and bacterial vaccines are required in order to "boost" and extend protection.

Critics of the mass vaccination system point to the fact that before many vaccines were introduced in the early 1900's, deaths and injuries from childhood diseases in technologically advanced countries such as the U.S. were already on a steep decline because of better sanitation, nutrition and health care. Although vaccination has been credited with eradicating smallpox from the world and eliminating polio from the western hemisphere, there is a scientific question as to whether vaccines can eradicate all of the viruses and bacteria for which we vaccinate, no matter how many booster doses of vaccines are given. Some viruses and bacteria that cause disease in humans also live in animals and some viruses and bacteria are very adaptable and can change their character in order to survive (an example is the way some bacteria have changed their character and become resistant to penicillin and other antibiotics). This may have been the case in the late 1980's when, after two decades of measles vaccination in the U.S., a more virulent type of measles was seen in an outbreak among American children and adults.

Because few scientific studies have been conducted to define the biological mechanism of how vaccines work in the body at the cellular and molecular level, there are no pathological profiles to describe the biological mechanism of vaccine injury and death. Therefore, doctors do not have lab tests or pathological markers to distinguish vaccine associated immune and neurological dysfunction from other causes of immune and neurological dysfunction. In addition, no well designed, long term studies have been conducted to find ways to identify and screen out high risk children or prove that giving as many as ten injections of viral and bacterial vaccines on one day is safe and effective.

With so many gaps in scientific knowledge about the long term effects of mass vaccination, there is growing concern that the mysterious rise in immune and neurological disorders during the past four decades, including learning disabilities, attention deficit disorder, asthma, autism, otitis media, diabetes, rheumatoid arthritis, lupus, multiple sclerosis, chronic fatigue immune deficiency syndrome, cancer and other chronic health problems may be caused in part by repeated manipulation of the immune system by giving multiple doses of viral and bacterial antigens in early childhood. It is unknown whether the use of a growing number of multiple viral and bacterial vaccines is weakening the human immune system or causing genetic change.

Proponents of mass vaccination, however, maintain that mass vaccination has eliminated most injuries and deaths associated with childhood infectious diseases. They maintain that, even when disease occurs in a person who has been vaccinated against it, the disease usually tends to be milder in vaccinated persons. But the primary achievement of mass vaccination, say proponents of mass vaccination, is the dramatic drop in the incidence of diseases for which vaccines have been developed and widely used in America. In 1945, there were more than 18,000 reported cases of diphtheria compared to less than 5 today; more than 13,000

27

reported cases of polio compared to about 10 today; more than 133,000 reported cases of pertussis compared to under 10,000 today; and 346 reported cases of smallpox compared to none today. The significant reduction in health care costs associated with treating infectious childhood diseases is also cited as compelling evidence that mass vaccination is a cost effective public health measure.

Chapter Five

HOW VACCINES ARE MADE

F ollowing is a general overview of how different vaccines are produced. Each manufacturer has patented a unique method for production. The following information is broadly representative of common production methods

DPT VACCINE: DPT vaccine is an inactivated bacterial vaccine. To produce the pertussis vaccine portion of the DPT vaccine, whole B. pertussis bacteria are grown in a modified Cohen-Wheeler broth, harvested, inactivated through heat and chemical treatments and suspended in a solution containing such chemicals as potassium phosphate, sodium chloride and thimerosal (mercury), which is used as a preservative. Aluminum is added as an adjuvant. The pertussis vaccine is then combined with the DT vaccine.

DT VACCINE: The diphtheria and tetanus toxoid are detoxified by use of formaldehyde and diluted with a solution containing such chemicals as sodium phosphate, glycine and thimerosal as a preservative. Aluminum is added as an adjuvant.

DTaP VACCINE: Unlike the DPT vaccine, the purified acellular or DTaP vaccine does not contain the whole B. pertussis bacteria. DTaP vaccine is made by separating out and removing many of the toxins in the whole B. pertussis bacteria and only using a few components of the bacteria in the vaccine. These remaining components, including pertussis toxin, may be detoxified by using formaldehyde. Thimerosal is usually added as a preservative and aluminum added as an adjuvant. The acellular pertussis vaccine is then combined with the DT vaccine.

MMR VACCINE: MMR vaccine used in the U.S. is a live virus vaccine. It contains (1) a weakened (partially inactivated) live measles virus derived from Enders' attenuated Edmonston strain and grown in cell cultures of chick embryo; (2) a weakened live strain of mumps virus grown in cell cultures of chick embryo; and (3) a weakened Wistar RA 27/3 strain of live attenuated rubella virus grown in human diploid cell (W-38) culture originating from the tissues of a fetus aborted in 1964 after the mother was infected with rubella. There is no preservative. MMR vaccine contains the antibiotic neomycin. Sorbitol and hydrolyzed gelatin are added as stabilizers.

29

The live virus measles vaccine, mumps vaccine and rubella vaccine are also available as single vaccines but most often doctors give these vaccines as the MMR vaccine unless single antigens are specifically requested.

LIVE ORAL POLIO VACCINE (OPV): The live oral polio vaccine used in the U.S. is a mixture of three types of attenuated (weakened or partially inactivated) polioviruses which have been grown in African green monkey kidney cell culture. The cells are then grown in a medium consisting of a salt solution containing amino acids, antibiotics and calf serum. After cell growth, the medium is removed and replaced with a medium containing the virus but no calf serum. The vaccine contains sorbitol and the antibiotics streptomycin and neomycin.

INACTIVATED POLIO VACCINE (IPV): The inactivated poliovirus vaccine used in the U.S. is a sterile suspension of three types of poliovirus grown in cultures of VERO cells, a continuous line of African green monkey kidney cells. The viruses are concentrated, purified and made noninfectious by inactivation with formaldehyde. IPV vaccine contains phenoxyethanol and formaldehyde as preservatives and the antibiotics neomycin, streptomycin and polymyxin. An IPV vaccine using human diploid cell cultures, rather than monkey kidney cell cultures, is used in some other countries.

HAEMOPHILUS INFLUENZA B VACCINE (HIB): Haemophilus influenza type b vaccine used in the U.S. today is a polysaccharide conjugate vaccine. It does not contain the HIB bacteria, just the organism's capsular polysaccharide. The vaccine is a sterile solution of a conjugate of oligosaccharides of the capsular antigen of Haemophilus influenza type b and diphtheria protein dissolved in sodium chloride.

HEPATITIS B VACCINE: The first hepatitis B virus vaccines developed in the 1970's were made using virus isolated from the blood of human chronic hepatitis B carriers. A plasma-derived hepatitis B vaccine was licensed by the U.S. in 1981 and used in high risk populations in the 1980's until a genetically engineered, recombinant hepatitis B vaccine was developed.

Today, hepatitis B recombinant vaccine used in the U.S. is derived from hepatitis B surface antigens produced in yeast cells. A portion of the hepatitis B virus gene is cloned into the yeast (a common baker's yeast) and the vaccine is produced from cultures of this recombinant yeast strain. The vaccine is treated with formaldehyde and contains 95 percent hepatitis B virus surface antigen, 4 percent yeast protein, aluminum hydroxide and thimerosal added as a preservative.

VARICELLA ZOSTER (CHICKEN POX) VACCINE: Chicken pox vaccine is made from the Oka/Merck strain of live attenuated (weakened) varicella virus. The virus was initially obtained from a child with natural varicella, introduced into human embryonic lung cell cultures, adapted to and propagated in embryonic guinea pig cell cultures and finally propagated in human diploid cell cultures. The vaccine contains sucrose, phosphate, glutamate and processed gelatin as stabilizers.

Chapter Six

REACTIONS TO VACCINES

Although many individuals do not experience serious reactions after vaccination, an unknown number of others do. Between 12,000 and 14,000 reports of hospitalizations, injuries and deaths are reported every year to the federal Vaccine Adverse Event Reporting System (VAERS). It is estimated that these reports represent, at best, only 10 percent of all adverse events which occur following vaccination because less than 10 percent of all physicians will report health problems patients experience following vaccination. There is little follow-up conducted by the government of serious events which are reported following vaccination to determine how many of these events are, in fact, caused by vaccinations. Therefore, there are no accurate statistics for estimating how many deaths and long term health problems are caused by vaccinations every year in the U.S.

Although different batches of DPT vaccine can vary widely in terms of how many B. pertussis organisms are in the batch (and therefore, how much pertussis toxin, endotoxin and other kinds of toxins are in the batch), and, although some lots of DPT vaccine can be associated with higher numbers of reports of hospitalizations, injuries and deaths than other lots, the Food and Drug Administration does not recall lots of DPT vaccine from the market.

Although too little scientific study has been conducted to explain why some children have serious vaccine reactions within hours, days or weeks following vaccination and others do not, it is thought to be due to a combination of factors including:

(1) the **general health of the child** at the time of vaccination;
(2) **genetic predisposition**;
(3) whether there are **identifiable high risk factors** such as a history of previous reactions;
(4) the **type of vaccine**(s) given;
(5) **vaccine lot variability**

Adverse reactions to vaccines can range from very mild to severe and can result in temporary discomfort, such as fever or sore leg, to permanent damage including learning problems, behavior disorders, mild to severe mental retardation, uncontrollable seizures and paralysis. The most extreme result of a vaccine reaction is death, which can occur within a few minutes from a sudden allergic reaction or within days, weeks, months or years after the vaccination, depending upon the vaccine and the individual.

DOCTORS MUST KEEP RECORDS AND PROVIDE INFORMATION:

The chance of having a serious reaction and suffering permanent damage after receiving one or more vaccines may or may not be statistically small depending upon the vaccine and what is known about it. With the exception of DPT vaccine, few studies have been conducted to determine rates of reactions to most vaccines we use and no large, long term studies have been conducted to evaluate the effects of multiple vaccination on the American population or to compare the health over time of vaccinated individuals to unvaccinated individuals.

When it happens to you or your child, the risks are 100%. Therefore, it is important to remember that federal law requires that a health care provider, who administers vaccine, must keep a permanent record of the vaccine manufacturer's name and lot number. The law also requires that you be provided with information about benefits and risks of the vaccine you or your child will receive before it is administered. This information should include instructions about how to monitor for possible adverse reactions following vaccination.

Chapter Seven

HEALTH PROBLEMS ASSOCIATED WITH VACCINES

T he following section will review the kinds of health problems, both acute and long term that have been associated with different childhood vaccines. Some of these health problems have compelling scientific evidence that they are causally related to vaccination. For the majority, not enough credible scientific study has been conducted to make a determination either way. It is important to remember that, because so much is still unknown about the effects of viral and bacterial vaccines on the human body, ALL significant health problems that occur following vaccination should be immediately investigated by a doctor, written down in the medical records and reported to the Vaccine Adverse Event Reporting System (VAERS). You can also obtain a questionnaire from NVIC to register a vaccine reaction in NVIC's Vaccine Adverse Event Registry, which is serving as a database for scientific evaluation and future reports (see information in Chapter 12).

For more detailed descriptions of DPT vaccine reactions contained in case histories, many of them first-hand descriptions by parents whose children have been injured or killed by vaccines, you may want to refer to A Shot in the Dark (Coulter & Fisher, 1985, 1986, 1991) among the list of publications contained in the BIBLIOGRAPHY at the end of this guide.

> REMINDER: There is a GLOSSARY OF MEDICAL TERMS at the end of this guide that describes health problems associated with diseases and vaccination. The GLOSSARY will help you identify vaccine reactions or a possible vaccine related health problem.

DPT VACCINE

The serious reactions most frequently reported to occur after DPT vaccination are prolonged crying for more than 3 hours; high pitched screaming; hypotonic/hyporesponsive or collapse/shock; fever over 103 F.; extreme lethargy (excessive sleepiness); and convulsions. A FDA/UCLA study published in 1981 concluded that 1 in 875 DPT shots is followed by a convulsion or collapse/shock.

Some children who suffer serious reactions to DPT vaccine go on to develop brain inflammation and permanent brain dysfunction. The British National Childhood Encephalopathy Study (NCES) which was the largest and most highly controlled study of brain damage in children ever conducted, found that 1 in 110,000 DPT shots results in a brain inflammation and 1 in 310,000 DPT shots results in permanent brain damage.

Other serious DPT reactions which have been reported include bulging fontanel (the soft spot on the newborn infant's head crown swells); cardiac and respiratory distress; apnea; Guillain-Barre syndrome; anaphylaxis; and mono and polyneuropathies. Other less serious reactions commonly reported are redness, pain, swelling and soreness at the injection site; rash; vomiting; diarrhea; loss of appetite; otitis media (inner ear infection) and respiratory infections.

Although the government and vaccine manufacturers have conducted studies which they say shows there is no association between DPT vaccine and sudden infant death syndrome (SIDS), there is evidence in the scientific literature and in the reports of infant deaths which occur following vaccine reactions that the DPT vaccine can cause infant death which is sometimes incorrectly misclassified as SIDS.

Because there has been little scientific study to explain the biological mechanism of vaccine death, no pathological profiles have been developed to make an accurate diagnosis or differentiate between vaccine-related deaths and infant deaths caused by other factors. Often when an infant dies following vaccination the death is classified as either SIDS or given another cause. Rarely will a coroner or doctor admit that a vaccine played any role in an infant's death. It is important for parents whose children who have died within 30 days of vaccination to make sure a report is made to the Vaccine Adverse Event Reporting System (VAERS). You can find out how to file a VAERS report at the end of this guide.

In 1991, a special committee of medical experts at the Institute of Medicine (IOM) issued a report that there is compelling scientific evidence that DPT vaccine can cause hypotonic/hyporesponsive episodes (also known as shock/collapse), protracted inconsolable crying, and acute brain inflammation (encephalopathy, encephalitis, encephalomyelitis). However, because too few scientific studies have ever been conducted to investigate DPT vaccine reactions, the 1991 IOM committee could not make a determination as to whether or not DPT vaccine can cause other serious health problems which are reported following DPT vaccination including aseptic meningitis; Guillain-Barre syndrome; hemolytic anemia; juvenile diabetes; learning disabilities; attention deficit disorder; peripheral mononeuropathy; thrombocytopenia or chronic neurological damage.

In 1994, another special committee of experts at the Institute of Medicine took a second look at the association between DPT vaccine and permanent brain damage. They reviewed the conclusions of a Ten Year Follow-Up of the landmark British National Childhood Encephalopathy Study (NCES), published in 1981, which investigated causes of brain injury in children. The NCES study defined chronic nervous system dysfunction (permanent brain damage) as "neurologic, behavioral, educational, motor, sensory, and self care dysfunctions," including residual seizure disorders.

This time, the IOM committee concluded that "some children who receive DPT and who experience a serious acute neurologic illness within 7 days thereafter would be expected to go on to experience chronic nervous system dysfunction or die." By the end of 1996, the federal vaccine injury compensation program created by The National Childhood Vaccine Injury Act of 1986 had made awards to nearly 1,000 vaccine victims and the majority of these awards were made for injuries or deaths caused by DPT vaccine.

During clinical trials held in the 1980's and early 1990's in Europe and the Third World, the efficacy of different DPT vaccines was found to range from 36 to 96 percent. In 1993, a whooping cough outbreak in Cincinnati revealed that more than 80 percent of the children under five who got whooping cough had been appropriately vaccinated for their age with DPT vaccine.

DTaP VACCINE

During clinical trials held in the 1980's and early 1990's in Europe and the Third World, the efficacy of DTaP vaccines was found to range from 82 to 96 percent. Reactions to DTaP were significantly less than for DPT.

The DtaP vaccine, which was licensed for use in infants in 1996, contains an acellular purified acellular pertussis vaccine. Most of the mild and serious reactions which have been reported following DPT vaccination have also been reported following DTaP vaccination, although it is thought that, because many toxins have been taken out of the pertussis portion of the vaccine, DTaP vaccine produces a fewer number of reactions.

A DTaP vaccine manufacturer product insert states that DTaP "has not been evaluated for carcinogenic, mutagenic potentials or impairment of fertility."

DT, Td and TETANUS VACCINE

The most common reactions reported to occur following DT vaccination include swelling and pain at the injection site; s eepiness; irritability; vomiting; loss of appetite; persistent crying; and fever. Paleness, cold skin, collapse, rash, and joint pain have also been reported.

In 1994 the Institute of Medicine concluded that there is compelling scientific evidence to conclude that tetanus, DT and Td vaccines can cause Guillain-Barre syndrome including death; brachial neuritis; and death from anaphylaxis (shock).

Because either no studies or too few scientific studies had ever been conducted to investigate tetanus, DT or Td reactions, a determination could not be made as to whether DT, Td or tetanus vaccine can cause other serious health problems which are reported following tetanus, DT and Td vaccination including residual seizure disorders, demyelinating diseases of the central nervous system (transverse myelitis, optic neuritis and acute disseminated encephalomyelitis), peripheral mononeuropathy, arthritis, and erythema multiforme (lesions of the skin or mucous membranes).

Vaccine makers state that tetanus, DT and Td vaccine provides protection for at least ten years after three or four "primary series"' doses have been given.

MMR VACCINE

The most frequent reactions reported to occur following MMR vaccination include brief burning and stinging at the injection site, fatigue, sore throat, cough, runny nose, headache, dizziness, fever, rash, nausea, vomiting or diarrhea, and sore lymph glands. Other reported reactions include anaphylaxis, convulsions, encephalopathy, otitis media, conjunctivitis, nerve deafness, thrombocytopenia purpura, optic neuritis, retinitis, arthritis, Guillain-Barre syndrome, and subacute sclerosing panencephalitis.

In 1981, the British National Childhood Encephalopathy Study concluded that there was a statistically significant association between measles vaccination and the onset of a serious neurological disorder within 14 days of receiving measles vaccine. The risk for previously normal children was estimated to be 1 in 87,000 measles vaccinations.

In 1991, the Institute of Medicine concluded that there is compelling scientific evidence that the rubella vaccine portion of the MMR shot can cause acute arthritis, with the highest incidence occurring in adult women who receive rubella vaccine (up to 15 percent) and that some individuals go on to develop chronic arthritis. Because either no studies or too few scientific studies have ever been conducted to investigate rubella vaccine reactions, a determination could not be made as to whether rubella vaccine causes other serious health problems which have been reported following rubella vaccination including thrombocytopenia purpura, radiculoneuritis (spinal nerve pain) or other neuropathies such as carpal tunnel syndrome.

In 1994, the Institute of Medicine concluded that there is compelling scientific evidence that the measles vaccine and the MMR vaccine can cause anaphylaxis that can end in death and that the MMR vaccine can cause thrombocytopenia (a decrease in the number of platelets, the cells involved in blood clotting) that can end in death. The incidence of thrombocytopenia was estimated to be 1 case per 30,000 to 40,000 vaccinated children. The IOM also concluded that the measles vaccine portion of the MMR vaccine can cause vaccine-strain measles virus infection that can end in death.

Because either no studies or too few studies have ever been conducted to investigate MMR vaccine reactions, a determination could not be made as to whether measles or mumps vaccine causes encephalitis or encephalopathy (brain disease); sensorineural deafness, or insulin dependent diabetes mellitus; whether the mumps vaccine causes aseptic meningitis, orchitis (inflammation of the testis) or sterility; or whether the measles vaccine causes subacute sclerosing panencephalitis, residual seizure disorders, optic neuritis, transverse myelitis, or Guillain-Barre syndrome.

In 1995, a British study concluded that adults who were vaccinated with measles vaccine as children were at much higher risk of developing inflammatory bowel disease, such as Crohn's disease and ulcerative colitis, as adults. Several researchers are looking into the possible link between inflammatory bowel disease and measles vaccine as well as other vaccines.

The vaccine manufacturer's product insert for MMR vaccine states "It is also not known whether [the vaccine] can cause fetal harm when administered to a pregnant woman or can affect reproduction capacity" and "it is not known whether measles or mumps vaccine virus is secreted in human milk. Recent studies have shown that lactating postpartum women immunized with live attenuated rubella vaccine may secrete the virus in breast milk and transmit it to breast-fed infants."

An MMR vaccine manufacturer states that in a study of 279 children 11 months to 7 years of age, MMR vaccine was shown to be 95 to 99 percent effective. Protection is estimated to persist for up to 11 years. In a measles outbreak in the U.S. in the late 1980's and early 1990's, it was found that there were a significant number of vaccine failures in older children, teenagers and adults, when the disease can be more severe. The government proceeded to recommend that a second MMR shot be given to boost immunity either before entrance to kindergarten or before entrance to junior high school.

In the national outbreak of measles during the late 1980's and early 1990's, it also became apparent that children who had been vaccinated before 15 months of age were also at risk for vaccine failure, especially if

39

their mothers had recovered naturally from measles disease as children. An MMR vaccine manufacturer states "Infants who are less than 15 months of age may fail to respond to the measles component of the vaccine due to presence in the circulation of residual measles antibody of maternal origin, the younger the infant, the lower the likelihood of seroconversion." The manufacturer goes on to advise that infants vaccinated at less than 12 months of age will have to be revaccinated after 15 months of age even though "there is some evidence to suggest that infants immunized at less than one year of age may not develop sustained antibody levels when later reimmunized."

The measles outbreaks in the late 1980's and early 1990's in the U.S. also demonstrated that babies, whose young vaccinated mothers had never naturally recovered from measles infection as children, were vulnerable to measles infection from birth. The young vaccinated mothers did not have natural maternal antibodies to transfer to their newborns to protect them from measles in the first year of life. In the 1989-91 measles outbreak in the U.S., the largest increase in measles cases was in infants under one year old.

In 1995, there were 309 cases of measles reported in the U.S.. Out of 219 cases where vaccination status was known, 123 (56 percent) had been vaccinated with at least one dose. Of 285 measles cases where age was known, 38 percent were under 5 years old and 39% were more than 20 years old.

NOTE: In 1995 and 1996, reports of an association between autism and vaccination (specifically suggesting a possible link with MMR vaccine) surfaced and is currently being explored by parents and researchers. If you would like to obtain more information on vaccination and autism, you can order a special *AUTISM AND VACCINES* information packet from NVIC.

POLIO VACCINE

In 1994, the Institute of Medicine concluded that there is compelling scientific evidence that the live oral polio vaccine (OPV) can cause paralytic and nonparalytic polio that can end in death. The Centers for Disease Control estimated that the risk is 1 case of vaccine associated polio per 520,000 first OPV doses administered to an individual and 1 case per 12.3 million second or subsequent doses of OPV given to an individual. The IOM also concluded that the live oral polio vaccine can lead to vaccine strain poliovirus infection and death in individuals who come into close contact with those who have been recently vaccinated with OPV.

The live poliovirus lives in the gastrointestinal tract and is shed for 6 to 8 weeks in body wastes and in nose/throat secretions. The greatest risk for development of vaccine strain poliovirus infection is in immune compromised individuals but healthy children and adults can also be vulnerable for unknown reasons. The symptoms of vaccine associated polio are similar to that of polio disease and usually occur within two months of receiving the live vaccine or coming into contact with a vaccine recipient.

The IOM also concluded that there is compelling scientific evidence that OPV can cause Guillain-Barre syndrome (GBS), including death, and stated "the risk difference is approximately 2.5 per 100,000 people."

Because either no studies or too few studies have ever been conducted on polio vaccine reactions, a determination could not be made as to whether OPV causes transverse myelitis (spinal cord disease); whether inactivated polio vaccine (IPV) causes Guillain-Barre syndrome; or whether either OPV or IPV causes sudden infant death syndrome (SIDS).

A vaccine manufacturer's product insert for IPV states that "Long term studies ..... to evaluate carcinogenic potential or impairment of fertility have not been conducted." An IPV vaccine manufacturer also states in the product insert that, because participants in studies to evaluate adverse reactions to IPV were also given DPT vaccine simultaneously, "systemic reactions could not be attributed to a specific vaccine." Both OPV and IPV vaccine manufacturer's product inserts state that "It is also not known whether [the vaccine] can cause fetal harm when administered to a pregnant woman or can affect reproductive capacity."

An OPV vaccine manufacturer estimates that after three or more doses of OPV are given, protection will be induced in 90 percent or more of those vaccinated. An IPV vaccine manufacturer estimates that after three doses of IPV, protection will be induced in 97 to 100 percent of those vaccinated.

NOTE: In the 1990's, scientists in the U.S. and Europe began to culture monkey virus genes and protein out of patients suffering from immune and neurological dysfunction and those dying from rare bone, lung and brain cancers. Because both inactivated and live polio vaccines have been grown on the kidney tissues of monkeys, some of these scientists have concluded that polio vaccines contaminated with monkey viruses have infected an unknown number of humans and may be passed from parent to child. One California microbiologist has presented evidence that the HIV-1 virus may be a monkey-human genetic hybrid created when humans got experimental polio vaccines contaminated with monkey viruses. Another California pathologist has cultured out cytomegalovirus fragments from patients suffering from immune and neurological dysfunction, including chronic fatigue syndrome and psychological disorders and genetically traced the virus back to the African green monkey, which is used to produce the live polio vaccine. If you would like to learn more about contaminated polio vaccines, you can order a special *POLIO VACCINE CONTAMINATION* information packet from NVIC.

HAEMOPHILUS INFLUENZA TYPE B VACCINE (HIB)

Reported common reactions to Hib vaccine include fever and pain and swelling at injection site. Rash, hives, irritability, restless sleep, prolonged crying, diarrhea, vomiting, loss of appetite, convulsions, collapse/shock, and Guillain-Barre syndrome have also been reported. Some of the studies used to evaluate the reactivity of Hib vaccine were complicated by the fact that Hib vaccine was given simultaneously with DPT and OPV vaccine. Today, most children receive a DPTH combination shot containing DPT and Hib vaccine in one shot. When a reaction occurs, it is difficult to determine which of the four vaccines in the shot were responsible for the reaction.

In 1994, the Institute of Medicine concluded that there is compelling scientific evidence that vaccination with earlier versions of the Hib vaccine, unconjugated PRP Hib vaccines, resulted in early onset of Hib disease in children over 18 months of age. Apparently, the early Hib vaccines caused children, who had been recently vaccinated, to be more vulnerable to becoming infected with Hib disease for at least 7 days after vaccination.

The newer conjugate Hib vaccines now being used are thought to be more quickly effective, leaving children less vulnerable to Hib disease shortly after vaccination. However, the IOM report stated that "Because immunization with Hib vaccines may lead to a transient decrease in protective antibody levels, unimmunized children at increased risk of colonization (household or day-care contact with individuals with recent cases of Hib infection) may require special [protective] measures." One Hib vaccine manufacturer states "There have been rare reports to the Vaccine Adverse Events Reporting System (VAERS) of Hib disease following full primary immunization."

Because either no studies or too few studies have ever been conducted to investigate Hib vaccine reactions, the IOM could not make a determination about whether Hib vaccine causes transverse myelitis, Guillain-Barre syndrome, thrombocytopenia, anaphylaxis or sudden infant death syndrome.

A manufacturer of HIB vaccine states in the product insert that the vaccine "has not been evaluated for its carcinogenic, mutagenic potential or impairment of fertility" and "it is also not known whether [the vaccine] can cause fetal harm when administered to a pregnant woman or can affect reproduction capacity."

In 1995, out of 74 Hib disease cases where age and vaccination status were known, 41 or 55 percent had received at least one Hib shot; 22 were appropriately vaccinated for their age; and 18 had completed the primary series.

HEPATITIS B VACCINE

A hepatitis B vaccine manufacturer's studies found that injection site and systemic complaints were reported following up to 17 percent of all hepatitis B injections. Reactions, which are reported to occur following more than 1 percent of hepatitis B injections, include soreness, pain and swelling at the site of the injection; fatigue and weakness; headache; fever of more than 100 F.; nausea; diarrhea; throat and upper respiratory infection; sweating; body aching; lightheadedness; chills; vomiting; abdominal pain/cramps; loss of appe-

43

tite; rhinitis; influenza; cough; vertigo/dizziness; rash; hives; arthritis/arthralgia including joint, back, neck and shoulder pain; neck stiffness; swollen lymph nodes; insomnia; earache and hypotension.

Other reactions that have been reported following hepatitis B vaccine include anaphylactic symptoms within a few hours of vaccination; peripheral neuropathy including Bell's Palsy; muscle weakness; Guillain-Barre syndrome; optic neuritis; tinnitus; neurological disorders such as transverse myelitis; herpes zoster; thrombocytopenia and visual disturbances. A hepatitis B vaccine manufacturer states that "an apparent hypersensitivity syndrome (serum-sickness-like) of delayed onset has been reported days to weeks after vaccination including arthralgia/arthritis (usually transient), fever and dermatologic reactions such as urticaria, erythema multiforme."

In 1994, the Institute of Medicine reported that there is compelling scientific evidence to conclude that the hepatitis B vaccine causes shock (anaphylaxis). Because either no studies or too few studies have ever been conducted to investigate hepatitis B reactions, a determination could not be made as to whether or not hepatitis B vaccine causes Guillain-Barre syndrome; central demyelinating diseases such as transverse myelitis, optic neuritis or multiple sclerosis; acute or chronic arthropathy (joint disease); or sudden infant death syndrome.

A hepatitis B vaccine manufacturer states in the product insert that "it is also not known whether the vaccine can cause fetal harm when administered to a pregnant woman or can affect reproduction capacity" and "it is not known whether the vaccine is excreted in human milk. Because many drugs are excreted in human milk, caution should be exercised when the vaccine is administered to a nursing woman."

A hepatitis B vaccine manufacturer states that after three doses of hepatitis B vaccine, 94 to 98 percent of adults 20 to 40 years old and 89 percent over 40 years old are protected. Efficacy for children after three doses is estimated at 96 to 99 percent. The manufacturer states that "the duration of protective effect in healthy vaccinees is unknown at present and the need for booster doses is not yet defined." There is concern among some scientists that babies vaccinated with hepatitis B vaccine will have waning immunity as teenagers and adults when they would be more likely to contract hepatitis B disease.

VARICELLA ZOSTER (CHICKEN POX) VACCINE

Reactions which have been most frequently reported after varicella zoster vaccination include, pain, soreness and swelling at injection site; chicken pox rash at injection site; chicken pox lesions on the body within 1 to 4 weeks of vaccination; and fever over 102 degrees F. Other reported reactions include upper respiratory infection; cough; irritability/nervousness; fatigue; disturbed sleep; diarrhea; loss of appetite; vomiting; otitis media; headache; abdominal pain; nausea; swollen lymph glands; hives; arthralgia; pneumonitis; and febrile seizures.

A varicella zoster vaccine manufacturer states in the product insert:

● "Individuals vaccinated with [the vaccine] may potentially be capable of transmitting the vaccine virus to close contacts. Therefore, vaccine recipients should avoid close association with susceptible high risk individuals (e.g., newborns, pregnant women, immunocompromised persons);"

● "It is also not known whether [the vaccine] can cause fetal harm when administered to a pregnant woman or can affect reproduction capacity" and "it is not known whether varicella vaccine virus is secreted in human milk. Therefore, because some viruses are secreted in human milk, caution should be exercised if [the vaccine] is administered to a nursing woman;"

● "[the vaccine] has not been evaluated for its carcinogenic or mutagenic potential, or its potential to impair fertility;"

● "There are no data relating to simultaneous administration of [the vaccine] with DTP or OPV."

Efficacy rates for chicken pox vaccine, licensed in the U.S. in 1995, have not been reliably established but are thought to be between 70 to 90 percent against infection for 7 to 10 years after vaccination. The vaccine is not effective in children under 12 months old and so t is recommended for children over one year old. In all pre-licensure clinical trials, some vaccinated children came down with chicken pox but were reported to have had relatively few lesions and a milder course of the disease. A varicella zoster vaccine manufacturer states that "the duration of protection is unknown at present and the need for booster doses is not defined."

The death rate for chicken pox is 1.4 per 100,000 cases in healthy children but rises to nearly 31 per 100,000 cases in adults. There is concern among some doctors that mass vaccination with chicken pox vaccine will drive the disease out of the normal childhood population, where it is mild for most children, into the infant and adult populations where it can be more dangerous. The vaccine's questionable rate of efficacy may contribute to cases occurring in these more vulnerable age groups in the future.

There is also concern that injecting children with a live virus varicella zoster vaccine may cause the vaccine virus to lay dormant in the body and be reactivated later in life in the form of herpes zoster (shingles). A varicella zoster vaccine manufacturer states that "the long term effect on the incidence of herpes zoster, particularly in those vaccinees exposed to natural varicella, is unknown at present."

Chapter Eight

BEFORE YOUR CHILD IS VACCINATED

One of the most important purposes of this information guide is to help parents, who have made the decision to vaccinate with one or more vaccines, to try to minimize vaccine reactions and become a more effective partner with a physician in making an educated vaccination decision for a child. Following are several steps that can be taken if you choose to vaccinate your child:

1. **PHYSICAL EXAM**: Ask your doctor to give your child a careful physical exam before each vaccination to determine that your child is in good health and there is no illness, especially fever at the time of vaccination. (Make sure the results of the exam are written in your child's medical record so that you have proof of the state of health your child was in before vaccination). Be sure to tell your doctor if your child has recently recovered from an illness or if any other members of your family are ill. Some scientific literature suggests that not only is an individual at increased risk of reacting to a vaccination if there is a coinciding viral or bacterial illness, but also an ill individual may not mount the expected antibody response to the vaccination.

Precaution: In order to help achieve a 100% vaccination rate in the U.S., the current federal government recommendation is to vaccinate children at every opportunity including emergency room visits or hospitalization. Doctors are being encouraged to screen children for their vaccination status when accompanying parents or siblings for other services. Health care providers in subspecialty clinics (for example, cancer clinics) are also being encouraged to screen patients for missed vaccinations.

It is common for hospital and clinic or emergency room staff to ask you about your child's vaccination status. You don't have to provide them with written proof. A verbal answer is satisfactory. However, if you are being questioned closely and feel that you are being pressured into vaccinating your sick child without your consent, you should understand that you have the right to refuse to give permission to have your sick child vaccinated if you believe vaccination at the time will endanger your child's health or life. You may choose to reassure medical personnel that you will consult a private pediatrician for further guidance about vaccination.

Special Precaution: When pregnant women are admitted to a hospital to have a baby, many times while in active labor, the hospital will require that the mother or father sign a paper agreeing to have the baby treated by medical personnel while in the hospital. Signing this paper may also constitute your consent to have your newborn vaccinated with hepatitis B vaccine shortly after birth. Many parents have reported that their newborns are being vaccinated without their knowledge and, when they ask why, they are told they signed a consent form prior to admission agreeing to medical treatment the hospital determined was necessary. Read any consent form you sign carefully. If you do not want your newborn vaccinated shortly after birth, you have the right to sign it after writing in an exception, such as, "I do not consent to have my child given any vaccinations prior to discharge from the hospital." Bring this to the attention of the person admitting you and the nursery supervisor and ask to have it printed on the outside of your chart. Some parents take the extra precaution of not leaving the newborn alone with hospital personnel without being able to observe the baby.

2. **DETAILED MEDICAL HISTORY**: The examining physician should take and record a detailed medical history of your child and your family (parents, grandparents, uncles and cousins) before the child is vaccinated. Be sure to mention if your child or anyone in your family has a history of convulsions or neurologic disease, severe allergies, immune system disorders or a history of reactions to vaccinations. Don't forget to tell your doctor if your child was born prematurely, had a difficult labor and delivery, is chronically ill or has breathing problems. Most importantly, be sure to tell your doctor about any previous vaccine reactions. Don't leave anything out of your description of the way your child reacted (or did not react) to a previous vaccination. Usually the appointment is too short for the doctor to ask everything, so it is a good idea prior to your appointment to take a few minutes and write down your child's medical history. Ask to have a copy placed in your child's medical record.

3. **THE TIMING OF VACCINATION**: Historically, Japan has not routinely given pertussis vaccine to children under the age of two years and some European countries have not routinely vaccinated children until three to six months of age. Some doctors maintain that a child's immature immune and neurological systems, which develop most rapidly within the

first few years of life, are also most vulnerable to insult in the first few years of life. Others believe that it is important to wait to determine whether a newborn has an underlying neurological or immune system disorder or other undiagnosed health problems before vaccination begins.

Some parents, who have made the decision to vaccinate, are choosing to begin vaccination at a later age and are taking special precautions to keep their unvaccinated children out of daycare or crowds to reduce the risk of exposing their children to adults and other children who may be sick with serious diseases. Many parents, who have decided to either delay vaccination or who have decided not to vaccinate, are consulting health care professionals who specialize in chiropractic, homeopathic, naturopathic, Traditional Chinese Medicine (including acupuncture) and other holistic health care therapies which focus on enhancing the functioning of the immune system and maintaining wellness.

Other parents, however, especially those with children in daycare, are choosing to begin vaccinating early but are allowing only one or two different vaccinations to be given simultaneously rather than three or four at a time. Some parents are choosing to space vaccinations further apart so that, if a reaction occurs, there is less confusion about which vaccine may have caused the reaction. These parents also feel more comfortable with allowing more time between vaccinations to give the child's immune system extra time to adjust to the viral and bacterial antigens that have been introduced.

Because U.S. federal vaccine policy today allows a one-year old child to be vaccinated with as many as 10 different viral and bacterial vaccines on one day, you should consider whether you want your child to get just one or two vaccines or many different vaccines on one day. Whatever option you choose, becoming better informed about your options will make you more comfortable with your decision.

4. **ON THE DAY OF VACCINATION**: Some physicians suggest a child should be given fruit juice or glucose water before and after a DPT shot to help maintain blood sugar levels and be given fever controlling medicines such as Tylenol. Some medical literature suggests that Vitamin C deficiency may play a role in severe reactions to vaccination and some parents supplement their child's diet with vitamin C before vaccination.

None of these measures, however, will guarantee that your child will not have a vaccine reaction. You might want to consider having your child vaccinated in the morning in order to have a long period of time during the day to observe your child following the shot.

5. **CHECK THE VIAL AND KEEP RECORDS**: Whenever your child receives a vaccination, it is a good idea to check the vial of vaccine to make sure it is the type of vaccine you have agreed to give your child and that the expiration date on the vial has not expired. You may want to consider asking for a new, unopened vial of vaccine if you suspect the vial has been stored for some time and your child would be receiving the last dose in the vial.

A parent should always ask for their own personal copy of the vaccination record to keep in a file at home. This record should include the type of vaccine, date and lot numbers.

BEFORE YOU VACCINATE, ASK EIGHT:

1. Is my child sick right now?

2. Has my child had a bad reaction to a vaccination before?

3. Does my child have a personal or family history of:

    - vaccine reactions
    - convulsions or neurological disorders
    - severe allergies
    - immune system disorders

4. Do I know if my child is at high risk of reacting?

5. Do I have full information on the vaccine's side effects?

6. Do I know how to identify a vaccine reaction?

7. Do I know how to report a vaccine reaction?

8. Do I know the vaccine manufacturer's name and lot number?

Chapter Nine

HEALTH CARE ALTERNATIVES

E very year, millions of Americans consult health care professionals who provide therapies designed to enhance the functioning of the immune system and help prevent disease as well as treat health problems. Chiropractic, homeopathic, naturopathic, Traditional Chinese Medicine (including acupuncture) and other non-allopathic health care options have been used both in the U.S. and around the world to assist in strengthening the body's natural ability to resist and cope with disease. These health care alternatives are gaining support among American consumers who want to maintain good health through making better nutrition and lifestyle choices and relying less upon synthetic drugs, vaccines and non-essential surgeries. Some parents of vaccine damaged children have reported that these non-allopathic therapies have helped to modify the severity of their children's vaccine injuries. As an informed health care consumer, you may want to become more educated about other disease prevention and treatment alternatives. Following is a list of organizations you may wish to contact for more information:

The following professional associations provide information and referrals to practitioners in your area:

The American Holistic Medical Association
4101 Lake Boone Trail #201
Raleigh, NC 27607 (include $5)
(919) 787-5181

World Chiropractic Alliance
2950 N. Dobson Road, Suite 1
Chandler, AZ 85224
1-800-347-1011

International Chiropractors Association
1110 North Glebe Rd, Suite 1000
Arlington, VA 22201
(703) 528-5000

International Chiropractic Pediatric Association
414 Ponce de Leon Ave.
Atlanta, Georgia 30308
404-872-5437

National Center for Homeopathy
801 N. Fairfax, Suite 306
Alexandria, VA 22314 (include $7)
(703) 548-7790

The American Association of Oriental Medicine
433 Front St.
Catasauqua, PA 18032
(610) 433-2448

American Association of Naturopathic Physicians
2366 Eastlake Ave., E. #322
Seattle, WA 98102 (include $5)
(206) 323-7610

Chapter Ten

CONTRAINDICATIONS TO VACCINATION

Most doctors follow the guidelines issued by the American Academy of Pediatrics (AAP) and the Centers for Disease Control (CDC) that define specific reasons for not giving a vaccine (contraindications). Because federal government health officials are trying to achieve a 100 percent vaccination rate in the U.S. with all recommended vaccines, these contraindications have become very narrow and explicit so that few individuals qualify for a medical exemption to vaccination.

The following **ABSOLUTE CONTRAINDICATIONS** to vaccination are based on information contained in the <u>Standards for Pediatric Immunization Practices</u>, which was published in 1993 by the U.S. Department of Health and Human Services (DHHS) and endorsed by the AAP and CDC, as well as the Februrary 7, 1992 supplement to the **MMWR** and the September 6, 1996 **MMWR** published by DHHS:

For all vaccines:

- anaphylactic (shock) reaction to a previous dose of a particular vaccine;

- anaphylactic (shock) reaction to a substance in a vaccine (such as neomycin in MMR vaccine);

- moderate or severe illness with or without a fever at the time of vaccination;

For DPT and DTaP Vaccine:

- encephalopathy (brain inflammation/disease) within seven days of a previous dose of DPT vaccine. *

* SIGNS OF ENCEPHALOPATHY COULD INCLUDE:

- <u>seizures</u> (such as repeated twitching, sudden jerking or stiffening of head, arms or legs; staring spells, sometimes accompanied by paleness and slight drooling; rolling of eyes back into or to the side of the head);

- <u>changes in levels of consciousness</u> (such as deep, prolonged sleep from which the child cannot be easily awakened, sometimes accompanied by cool or clammy skin and paleness)

- neurological signs (such as crossing of eyes, inability to suck or move an arm, leg or head; inability to recognize parents or respond to sound, touch or visual stimulation);

- sudden changes in behavior (such as uncontrollable crying or high pitched screaming; hyperactivity and inability to sleep alternating with deep sleep; unresponsiveness; or other severe changes in mental, emotional or physical behavior).

For Live Oral Polio Vaccine (OPV):

- if the person to be vaccinated has HIV infection (AIDS) or lives in a house with a person who has AIDS;

- if the person to be vaccinated has an immune system deficiency or is taking drugs or treatment which suppresses the immune system (such as cancer therapy) or lives in a house with such a person.

For Killed Inactivated Polio Vaccine (IPV):

- anaphylactic (shock) reaction to neomycin or streptomycin.

For Live MMR Vaccine:

- anaphylactic (shock) reaction to egg or neomycin;

- pregnancy (MMR, measles or rubella vaccine should not be given to women who are pregnant or who are considering becoming pregnant within the next 3 months);

- if the person to be vaccinated has an immune system deficiency or is on drugs or therapy that suppresses the immune system (such as cancer therapy).

For Live Monovalent Mumps Vaccine:

- pregnancy (mumps vaccine should not be given to women who are pregnant or who are considering becoming pregnant within the next 30 days).

The following conditions are considered *"PRECAUTIONS"* to vaccination by federal vaccine policymakers at the Centers for Disease Control and health care providers are directed to weigh the benefit and risks to an individual when deciding whether or not to vaccinate.

For the "P" or pertussis portion of DPT Vaccine:

- Fever of 105 F. or greater within 48 hours of a previous DPT shot (occurs 1 per 330 doses);

- Collapse or shock like state (hypotonic-hyporesponsive episode) within 48 hours of a previous DPT shot (occurs 1 per 1,750 doses);

- Seizures with or without fever within 72 hours of a previous DPT shot (occurs 1 per 1,750 doses);

- Persistent inconsolable crying lasting 3 hours or more within 48 hours of a previous DPT shot (occurs 1 per 100 doses).

* NOTE: In the past, the CDC and AAP have considered the above serious reactions to DPT vaccine, which they now list as "PRECAUTIONS," to be ABSOLUTE CONTRAINDICATIONS to further doses of pertussis vaccine. The NVIC has many documented cases of children who have reacted with either high fever, collapse/shock, seizures and persistent, uncontrollable crying or high pitched screaming to one or more DPT shots, and who have died or been severely brain damaged after being injected with more pertussis vaccine.

For OPV and IPV Vaccine:

- Pregnancy.

For MMR Vaccine:

- If the person to be vaccinated has received immunoglobulin (IG) within the past three months;

- If the person had an episode of thrombocytopenia within 6 weeks of an MMR shot.

- If the person has had an anaphylactic reaction to gelatin or gelatin-containing products.

With regard to *"PRECAUTIONS,"* the Standards for Pediatric Immunization Practices states: "The events or conditions listed as precautions, although not contraindications, should be carefully reviewed. The benefits and risks of administering a specific vaccine to an individual under the circumstances should be considered. If the risks are believed to out-weigh the benefits, the immunization should be withheld; if the benefits are believed to outweigh the risks (for example, during an outbreak or foreign travel), the immunizations should be given. Whether and when to administer DPT to children with proven or suspected underlying neuro-logic disorders should be decided on an individual basis. It is prudent on theoretical grounds to avoid vaccinating pregnant women. However, if immediate protection against poliomyelitis is needed, OPV, not IPV, is recommended."

THE STANDARDS FOR PEDIATRIC IMMUNIZATION PRACTICES AND CONTRAINDICATION GUIDELINES ISSUED BY THE CENTERS FOR DISEASE CONTROL ARE CONSIDERED BY SOME HEALTH EX-PERTS AND THE NATIONAL VACCINE INFORMATION CENTER TO BE A VERY RESTRICTED, MINIMUM LIST OF CONTRAINDICATIONS TO VACCINATION. There are other medical conditions and circumstances which may be reason to defer vaccination, which are not listed in the Standards for Pediatric Practices or in the CDC guidelines.

WHAT THE VACCINE MANUFACTURERS SAY

The product inserts published by the vaccine manufacturers contain more contraindications than listed by the Centers for Disease Control, Ameri-can Academy of Pediatrics or the Standards for Pediatric Immunization Practices. Drug companies selling vaccines are required by law to de-scribe and list adverse reactions and health problems associated with each vaccine they produce. Because these product inserts are periodi-cally updated, NVIC strongly urges all vaccine consumers to ask their doctor for a copy of the manufacturer's product insert to read *before* vac-cination takes place. Following are just a few of the specific contraindications listed by vaccine manufacturers in their product inserts:

For DPT Vaccine: "Hypersensitivity to any component of the vac-cine, including thimerosal, a mercury derivative, is a contraindication."...... "Routine immunization [with DPT] should be deferred during an outbreak of poliomyelitis...."..."The occurrence of any type of neurological symp-toms or signs, including one or more convulsions (seizures) following ad-ministration of this product is a contraindication to further use. Use of this product is also contraindicated if the child has a personal history of seizures. The presence of any evolving or changing disorder affecting the central nervous system is a contraindication to administration of DTP regardless of whether the suspected neurological disorder is associated with occurrence of seizure activity of any type."

For DTaP Vaccine: "Influenza virus vaccine should not be given within three days of the administration of [the vaccine]."

For MMR Vaccine: "Due caution should be employed in administration of MMR to persons with a history of cerebral injury, individual or family histories of convulsions, or any other condition in which stress due to fever should be avoided."

For OPV Vaccine: "Immunization should be deferred during the course of any febrile illness or acute infection. In addition, immunization should be deferred in the presence of persistent vomiting or diarrhea, or suspected gastroenteritis infection.".…"Prior to administration of the vaccine, the attending physician should warn or specifically direct personnel acting under their authority to convey the warnings to the vaccinee, parent, guardian or other responsible person of the possibility of vaccine-associated paralysis, particularly to the recipient, family members and other close personal contacts......The responsible adult should be informed of precautions to be taken such as handwashing after diaper changes."

For HIB Vaccine: "Hypersensitivity to any component of the vaccine, including diphtheria toxoid or thimerosal in the multidose presentation, is a contraindication."

For Varicella Zoster Vaccine: "Pregnancy should be avoided for three months following vaccination."......"Vaccine recipients should avoid use of salicylates [aspirin] for 6 weeks after vaccination with [the vaccine]....."

CDC "MISCONCEPTIONS" ARE NVIC PRECAUTIONS

At the end of the September 6, 1996 *MMWR,* the CDC lists "Misconceptions Concerning Contraindications to DTP." However, based on evidence in the medical literature; reports of injuries and deaths made by parents to NVIC; reports of hospitalizations, injuries and deaths made to the Vaccine Adverse Event Reporting System (VAERS); and other data collected by the Centers for Disease Control, the National Vaccine Information Center considers the following circumstances not to be "MISCONCEPTIONS" but to be significant GENERAL PRECAUTIONS to vaccination:

1. Soreness, redness or swelling at the vaccination site or temperature of less than 105 F.
2. Mild, acute illness with low-grade fever or mild diarrheal illness affecting an otherwise healthy child.
3. Current antibiotic therapy or the convalescent phase of an acute illness.
4. Recent exposure to an infectious illness.
5. Prematurity.
6. History of allergies or relatives with allergies.
7. Family history of convulsions. *
8. Family history of SIDS.
9. Family history of an adverse event following vaccination.

A Centers for Disease Control analysis in 1987 found that children who have a personal history of convulsions are nine times more likely to have a seizure following DPT vaccination and children who have a family history of convulsions are three times more likely to have a seizure following a DPT vaccination than children who do not have a personal or family history of convulsions.

ASK YOUR DOCTOR:

In addition to asking your doctor for a copy of the manufacturer's product insert, it is very important to consult other sources of information which may place an individual at increased risk for reacting to one or more vaccines. New research is being published and information is frequently being released concerning vaccines. Discuss your concerns with your doctor and ask questions. If you are not comfortable with the answers you are receiving or the way you are being treated, get a second or third opinion from a health care professional who respects your right to be an informed health care consumer.

Chapter Eleven

VACCINES AND THE LAW

T he following information on mandatory vaccination laws in different states for 1994-95 was published by the Centers for Disease Control:

- **Diphtheria, measles, rubella, polio vaccines**: Required by all 50 states;

- **Pertussis vaccine**: Required by all states except Idaho, Maine, Missouri, New York, Oregon, Pennsylvania, Texas and Washington;

- **Tetanus vaccine**: Required by all states except Missouri and New York;

- **Mumps vaccine:** Required by all states except Alaska, Arkansas, Iowa, Maryland, Missouri, New Mexico, Vermont and West Virginia.

- **Hib vaccine**: Varies, but most states require HIB for daycare and head start programs;

- **Hepatitis B vaccine:** Recommended in most states and legally required in about half the states.

Private schools and daycare centers as well as public schools and daycare centers are required to comply with state health regulations. In many states, the director of a private school is held responsible and can be fined if vaccination records are not current. Many colleges are requiring proof of vaccination for enrollment.

RECOMMENDATIONS VS. LAWS: It is important for you to know the legal requirements of the vaccination laws in your state and to understand the difference between a legal requirement and a recommendation. While vaccine policymakers in the AAP and CDC recommend that the MMR shot be given to all children, your state may legally require only measles and rubella vaccines. In this case, you have the legal option to vaccinate with only measles and rubella vaccines and not with mumps vaccine.

You also have the option in some states to be exempted from vaccination or re-vaccination if you can show proof of existing immunity. You can go to a private laboratory for a blood test to determine if there are enough antibodies to prove existing immunity to a disease such as measles or whooping cough. A blood test that measures antibody levels can cost $55 or more, depending on the disease.

While the CDC and AAP recommendations allow 10 different vaccines to be given on one day to a 12 month old child and most doctors give multiple vaccines simultaneously to children, it is not legally required by any state that this be done. You may have the legal right to choose at what age you want your child to be vaccinated and how many vaccines you want your child to receive on one day. For example, you may have the right to choose to have your doctor give your child a DPT and polio vaccination only on one day and return several months later for an MMR vaccination or other vaccines.

When making an informed vaccination decision, it is important to consider how age at the time of vaccination, as well as having many different viral and bacterial vaccines injected at once, may increase the risk of having a severe reaction as well as affect the ability of one or more vaccines to be effective.

LEGAL EXEMPTIONS TO VACCINATION

Religious, medical and philosophical exemptions are worded differently in each state. To use an exemption for your child, you must know specifically what the law says in your state. To obtain a copy of your law, ask your local reference librarian to help you. Ask for the public health codes, education and welfare laws pertaining to vaccination requirements for school entry.

When you become a member of the National Vaccine Information Center (NVIC), we will send you a summary of your state vaccination law upon request.

Philosophical Exemption: The following 17 states allow exemption to vaccination based on philosophical beliefs: **Arizona, California, Colorado, Idaho, Louisiana, Maine, Michigan, Minnesota, New Mexico, North Dakota, Ohio, Oklahoma, Rhode Island, Utah, Vermont, Washington and Wisconsin.**

In many of these states, individuals must object to all vaccines, not just a particular vaccine in order to use the philosophical objection or personal conviction exemption. Many state legislators are being urged by federal health officials and medical organizations to revoke this exemption to vaccination. If you are objecting to vaccination based on philosophical or personal conviction, keep an eye on your state legislature as public health officials seek to amend state laws to eliminate this exemption.

Religious Exemption: All states allow a religious exemption to vaccination except *Minnesota, Mississippi and West Virginia.*

The religious exemption is intended for people who possess a sincere religious belief against vaccination to the extent that if the state forced vaccination, it would be an infringement on their right to exercise their religious beliefs. Some state laws define religious exemptions broadly to include personal religious beliefs, similar to personal philosophical beliefs. Other states require an individual who claims a religious exemption to be a member of The First Church of Christ Scientist (Christian Science) or another bonafide religion whose written tenets include prohibition of invasive medical procedures such as vaccination. Some laws require a signed affidavit from the pastor of the church while others allow the parent to sign a notarized waiver. Prior to registering your child for school, you must check your state law to verify what proof may be needed.

Due to differences in state laws, the National Vaccine Information Center does not recommend or provide a prewritten waiver for religious exemption because it may not comply with what is required in your state, and may actually draw attention to your child, and you may be singled out and challenged.

If you are challenged, you could end up in litigation brought by your state or county health department to prove your religious beliefs. The religious exemption is granted based on the First Amendment to the Constitution, which is the right to freely exercise your religion. Because citizens are protected under the First Amendment of the United States, a state must have a "compelling State interest" before this right can be taken away. One "compelling State interest" is the spread of communicable diseases. In state court cases which have set precedent on this issue the freedom to act according to your own religious belief is subject to reasonable regulation with the justification that it must not threaten the welfare of society as a whole.

However, parents have successfully obtained religious exemptions to vaccination even when they do not belong to a church which has a written tenet prohibiting vaccination. The constitutional right to have and exercise personal religious beliefs, whether you are of the Christian, Jewish, Muslim or other faith, can be defended. If you exercise your right to religious exemption, you must be prepared to defend it. It is always best to define your personal religious beliefs against vaccination in your own words when you write a letter defending them. If you do belong to a church and take the time to educate the head of your local church about the sincerity of your personal religious beliefs regarding vaccination, obtaining a letter from your pastor, priest, rabbi or other spiritual counselor confirming your sincere religious beliefs may also be advisable.

Medical Exemptions: All 50 states allow medical exemption to vaccination. Most doctors follow the AAP and CDC guidelines. Proof of medical exemption must take the form of a signed statement by a Medical Doctor (M.D.) or Doctor of Osteopathy (D.O.) that the administering of one or more vaccines would be detrimental to the health of an individual. Most states do not allow Doctors of Chiropractic (D.C.) to write medical exemptions to vaccination.

Some states will accept a private physician's written exemption without question. Other states allow the state health department to review the doctor's exemption and revoke it if health department officials don't think the exemption is justified.

Proof of Immunity: Some states will allow exemptions to vaccination for certain diseases if proof of immunity can be shown to exist. Immunity can be proven if you or your child have had the natural disease or have been vaccinated. You have to check your state laws to determine which vaccines in your state can be exempted if proof of immunity is demonstrated.

Private medical laboratories can take blood (a titer test) and analyze it to measure the level of antibodies, for example, to measles or pertussis that are present in the blood. If the antibody level is high enough, according to accepted standards, you have obtained proof of immunity and may be able to use this for an exemption to vaccination.

Chapter Twelve

THE VACCINE INJURY COMPENSATION LAW AND REPORTING VACCINE REACTIONS

If you or your child suffered a reaction to a vaccination that caused an excess of $1,000 in medical bills or caused injuries that have lasted longer than six months, you may be entitled to benefits under the **National Childhood Vaccine Injury Act of 1986** (PL 99-660). This federal compensation system was created by Congress to provide reimbursement for medical and custodial care expenses or award a fixed amount in the case of a vaccine-related death. As of 1997, about 1,000 vaccine victims have received compensation totaling nearly $750 million.

Federal law also requires doctors or other health care professionals who give vaccines to:

• **REPORT ADVERSE EVENTS** (hospitalizations, injuries and deaths) occurring within 30 days of vaccination, including convulsions, shock, paralysis and other serious events, to the Vaccine Adverse Event Reporting System (VAERS). The doctor or other health care provider that administered the vaccination is not supposed to make a judgment as to whether the adverse event that occurred following vaccination was caused by the vaccine or not caused by the vaccine. The law says it is the duty of all vaccine administrators to report the event to the federal government *regardless* of whether they believe the vaccine caused the event.

Federal law also requires doctors or other health care providers who give vaccines to:

• **RECORD ADVERSE EVENTS** following vaccination in a person's permanent medical record;

• **KEEP A PERMANENT RECORD** of the date, manufacturer's name and lot number of all vaccinations given; and

• **PROVIDE INFORMATION** on vaccine benefits and risks BEFORE the vaccination is given either to the individual who will receive the vaccine or the parent or guardian of that individual.

If your doctor refuses to report a hospitalization, injury or death occurring within 30 days of a vaccination to VAERS, which is a violation of the federal law, you may want to consider filing a report of professional misconduct through your state medical licensing board.

If your doctor or health clinic won't report a serious event which occurred following a vaccination given to you or your child, you may report it by calling 1-800-822-7967 to receive a government Vaccine Adverse Event Report form. You should also report a death or severe reaction to the National Vaccine Information Center by calling (703) 938-DPT3 and asking for an NVIC Vaccine Adverse Event Registry questionnaire to be sent to you. Be sure to give your name, address, telephone number and brief description of what happened. You can also report a vaccine reaction to NVIC by accessing NVIC's website at http//www.909shot.com. By reporting to the NVIC, our organization can better monitor the effectiveness of the government's Vaccine Adverse Event Reporting System and gather important data on vaccine reactions for analysis that the government and vaccine manufacturers do not do.

Chapter Thirteen

THE NATIONAL VACCINE INFORMATION CENTER

You are ultimately responsible for the consequences of your health care choices and, therefore, it is very important to exercise your right to become fully informed about any medical procedure which you or your child undergoes, including vaccination. You can never become too knowledgeable about a disease or a medical procedure, such as vaccination, which carries a risk of injury or death and can affect your life or the life of your child.

The National Vaccine Information Center (NVIC), has existed since 1982 to provide the public with information about infectious diseases and vaccines. NVIC provides assistance to parents whose children have suffered vaccine reactions; promotes research to evaluate vaccine safety and effectiveness as well as to identify factors which place individuals at high risk for suffering vaccine reactions; and advocates the institution of oversight mechanisms within the mass vaccination system to make it safer.

NVIC's co-founders worked with federal legislators to help create the National Childhood Vaccine Injury Act of 1986 that set up a vaccine injury compensation program and included vaccine safety provisions such as mandatory reporting and recording of hospitalizations, injuries and deaths following vaccination. In 1989, the organization held an International Scientific Workshop to evaluate the neurological complications of pertussis and the pertussis vaccine. NVIC has provided information to more than 350,000 parents and health care providers since it was founded.

Advocating the right for citizens to make informed, independent vaccination decisions, NVIC represents you, the health care consumer, while serving as a consumer "watchdog" monitoring vaccine research, development, policymaking and legislation. As a charitable, consumer advocacy organization without grants from the government or major corporations, NVIC is entirely supported by individual donations from citizens to continue to do research and provide information to the public.

BECOME A MEMBER AND A NEWSLETTER SUBSCRIBER - We hope you have found this information helpful. NVIC also offers books, information packets, special reports, video and audiotapes and other information on diseases and vaccines. Please consider becoming a member of NVIC and subscribing to *THE VACCINE REACTION,* a bi-monthly newsletter which will bring you the latest news about the more than 200 vaccines being created; changes in state mandatory vaccination laws and state and federal vaccine policies; health care alternatives to vaccination; your right to informed consent to vaccination and many other vaccine-related issues.

Vaccination laws no longer pertain just to children, where mandatory vaccination laws in every state promote the policy of "no shots, no school." Many adult health care workers are required to get rubella, hepatitis B and other vaccines as a condition of employment. Most students cannot attend college without proof of vaccination. Parents are denied welfare benefits and food stamps if they cannot prove their children have received all the government-recommended vaccines. Many of the 200 vaccines being developed by drug companies and the government, including an AIDS vaccine, will be legally mandated to be used by children and adults. Stay up-to-date on what is happening and help secure your right to make informed health care choices.

To subscribe to *THE VACCINE REACTION* (send $18); to order the *Autism and Vaccination* information packet (send $15); to order the *Polio Vaccine Contamination* information packet (send $16); to order the 30-minute videotape *"The Other Side of the Story"* which includes general information on vaccines as well as interviews and footage of parents and their vaccine damaged children (send $20); or to get more information on how to become a member of NVIC, write to THE NATIONAL VACCINE INFORMATION CENTER, 512 W. Maple Ave., Suite 206, Vienna, VA 22180. To immediately order information, call 1-800-909-SHOT or access NVIC's website at www.909shot.com.

We thank you for your interest and hope that you will support NVIC's effort to prevent vaccine injuries and deaths through public education and win the right for all citizens to make informed vaccination choices for themselves and their children. Donations are gratefully accepted and your special donation will help NVIC continue to inform, represent and protect you, the health care consumer. All proceeds from this Guide directly support the work of NVIC.

GLOSSARY OF MEDICAL TERMS

AIDS (ACQUIRED IMMUNE DEFICIENCY SYNDROME) - A condition characterized by severe immune deficiency which leads to opportunistic infections, malignancies and neurologic lesions in individuals without a previous history of immune system dysfunction. AIDS is often associated with infection with HIV (human immunodeficiency virus). HIV-1 is a novel retrovirus which was not identified until the 1970's and is genetically similar to simian immunodeficiency virus (SIV), which is known to infect monkeys. Monkey tissues have historically been used to produce polio vaccines and other viral vaccines and some scientists maintain that HIV-1 may be a genetic monkey-human hybrid which was created when live viral vaccines contaminated with monkey viruses were used to produce vaccines. This theory is disputed by public health officials who have not been able to explain the origins of HIV or why many individuals infected with HIV go on to develop AIDS.

ANAPHYLAXIS (SHOCK) - Within minutes to 72 hours of vaccination, the following symptoms can occur: skin becomes very pale or body becomes flushed and starts to swell; skin breaks out in hives (mostly on the arms, legs and face, especially the eyes and lips) with intense itching; inability to breathe or wheezing (respiratory distress); throat swells shut and cuts off oxygen; nausea and vomiting with abdominal cramps; seizures; the heart can fail and end in death.

APNEA - A cessation of breathing for a few seconds to minutes, usually during sleep. Premature infants often have apnea spells, sometimes accompanied by slowing of the heartbeat (bradycardia) and bluish coloring of the skin due to lack of oxygen (cyanosis). Recurrent apnea spells can lead to respiratory distress and death. Apnea has been associated with sudden infant death syndrome (SIDS).

ARTHRALGIA - Mild or severe pain in a joint(s).

ARTHRITIS - Inflammation of a joint(s) with swelling, redness, stiffness, tenderness, and pain, especially during movement. Chronic inflammation of the joints that occurs with chronic arthritis can eventually lead to crippling of the body including fusion of the joints, deformed bones, compression of the spinal cord, the inability to move and severe, constant pain.

ASEPTIC MENINGITIS - An inflammation of the membranes covering the brain and spinal cord that is not caused by a bacterial infection. Usually caused by a viral infection, aseptic meningitis commonly begins with sudden flu-like symptoms including fatigue, fever, nausea and vomiting. Skin rashes may appear on the body. A severe headache in the front part of the head, stiffness of the neck when bending forward as well as stiffness of the spine are signs. Sometimes the person is very sleepy and slightly confused, but usually is rational and can function. Lung involvement may include sharp pains in the chest made worse by deep breathing or coughing. In the majority of cases, fever and other symptoms start to go away within 3 to 5 days and completely disappear in two weeks with full recovery. In unusually severe cases, the person is left with permanent muscular weakness and disability or the tendency to have recurrent attacks of aseptic meningitis.

ASTHMA - A disease of the airways characterized by hyperirritability of the bronchial tubes with widespread narrowing of the air passages. Asthma attacks cause paroxysms of wheezing, coughing, breathlessness and production of thick mucus. About one half of all cases of chronic asthma occur before age 10 and it has been estimated that up to 10 percent of all children in the U.S. suffer with asthma. The cause of asthma is not known but the disease is thought to be triggered by a reaction to substances in the environment, drugs, and foods, by infections or by strenuous exercise or emotional stress. The disease has traditionally been separated into two categories: *allergic asthma* which is thought to have an immunologic mechanism and involve genetic predisposition because it runs in families with histories of allergies; and *idiosyncratic asthma* which is thought to be "nonallergic." It is estimated that immunologic mechanisms are causally related to the development of asthma in 25 to 35 percent of all cases and play some role in another third of the cases. A variety of drugs have been used to treat the disease but nearly 50 percent of children still have asthma 10 years after the first episode. About 40 percent of all asthma sufferers are estimated to have milder attacks as they grow older. Rarely, an asthma attack can end in death.

ATTENTION DEFICIT DISORDER (ADD) - Inability to focus or sustain attention, with impulsive and hyperactive behavior. ADD is estimated to affect 5 to 10 percent of school-aged children and occurs in boys 10 times more frequently than in girls. ADD is usually diagnosed before age 7 years. Symptoms include distractibility; restlessness; difficulty concentrating for extended periods, especially without moving around; lack of organization; tendency to constantly shift from one activity to the next and become frustrated easily. There is no known cause and no consistently effective treatment, although millions of children with ADD have been placed on the drug Ritalin, which is not without significant side effects.

AUTISM - Also known as pervasive developmental disorder (PDD), this form of brain dysfunction is characterized by inability of the child to communicate and interact with others in a normal way. Autistic children often isolate themselves in their own world and refuse to make eye contact; have delayed speech; engage in obsessive repetitive movements such as spinning, tapping and flapping their hands and arms; cannot adapt to change in routine; and are unable to relate emotionally to others. Up to 30 percent of autistic children eventually develop seizure disorders. Many autistic children also have immune dysfunction including gastrointestinal problems, allergies, chronic ear and respiratory infections, and nutritional deficiencies.

BELL'S PALSY - Facial paralysis which occurs suddenly and is thought to involve swelling of the nerves. Although the precise cause is unknown, Bell's palsy is thought to be caused by a viral infection or immune system problem. Symptoms may begin with pain behind the ear followed by facial weakness and, within hours, can lead to partial or complete facial paralysis. Complete recovery within a few months occurs in many cases but some victims are left with permanent nerve damage including partial paralysis.

BRACHIAL NEURITIS - Inflammation of the nerve in the arm and shoulder which causes muscle weakness and a deep, steady, often severe aching in the shoulder and upper arm. Usually appears within 21 days of vaccination. As the pain subsides within days or weeks of appearing, weakness and atrophy (wasting, shrinking) of the arm and shoulder persist. Recovery is slow and may take up to 30 months.

CARPAL TUNNEL SYNDROME - A neuropathy of the median nerve at the wrist producing pain, tingling, numbness and weakness in the hands. Pain can radiate into the forearm, shoulder and neck.It is usually caused by repetitive motion, trauma, infection, and endocrine and autoimmune disorders.

CHRONIC FATIGUE SYNDROME (CFS) - Also known as chronic fatigue and immune dysfunction syndrome (CFIDS), myalgic encephalomyelitis, and "Yuppie Flu," Chronic Fatigue syndrome (CFS) is characterized by a wide range of immune and neurological system dysfunction including profound, chronic fatigue that can be disabling; joint and muscle pain and weakness; vision, balance and physical coordination problems; severe, chronic headaches; gastrointestinal symptoms; heart palpitations; inability to concentrate; loss of memory; deterioration of intellectual abilities; and personality changes. Lab tests often reveal high levels of Epstein-Barr virus antibodies and other signs indicating abnormal immune system functioning. Some sufferers also have abnormal brain scans revealing brain lesions. It is estimated that between one and two million Americans are suffering from CFS. Fewer than one-fifth of those who get CFS are estimated to recover completely with most patients being left with some chronic symptoms. Some CFS patients are totally disabled.

The cause of Chronic Fatigue syndrome is unknown, although some scientists theorize it is caused by an infectious virus that attacks the immune system and the brain. Others theorize that CFS is caused by a combination of factors including exposure to infectious agents and toxins as well as extreme physiological and psychological stress. The more than 70,000 Gulf War veterans who are reported to be suffering from "Gulf War syndrome" are exhibiting symptoms identical to CFS. (It is known that Gulf War veterans were given 17 different viral and bacterial vaccines, including experimental drugs and vaccines, before being exposed to environmental toxins in the Gulf War)

CONJUNCTIVITIS - Inflammation of the delicate membrane lining the eyelids and covering the eyeball usually caused by viruses, bacteria or allergies. The eyes are reddened, swollen, and discharge mucus secretions with itching and burning sensations.

CONVULSIONS (SEIZURES) - An involuntary contraction or series of contractions of the voluntary muscles due to disturbance of the electrical activity of the brain. Convulsions or seizures can be caused by infections, head trauma, metabolic disorders, high fevers, vaccine reactions and other conditions. A convulsion can occur only once or can be followed by the development of a permanent *residual seizure disorder* which involves recurring seizures. In children, the majority of seizures are diagnosed as being *idiopathic* - without a known cause.

There are a variety of different kinds of seizures including: *focal* seizures which occur predominantly on one side of the body and may affect only one arm or one leg; *generalized* convulsions which involve shaking, jerking, stiffness on both sides of the body; *tonic seizures* which are characterized by stiffness/rigidity; *petit mal* seizures in which there is sudden momentary loss of consciousness (for a few seconds or longer) characterized by blank staring without movement and may involve eye blinking or slight twitching; *grand mal* convulsions which usually start with loss of consciousness followed by violent jerking of the whole body for minutes or hours and, if not controlled, can lead to *status epilepticus* and death.

When individuals are having convulsions, they may have pale skin, drooling, rolling of the eyes back in the head or crossed eyes, make grunting sounds or other kinds of noises, lose bladder and bowel control, be unable to respond to sound or touch. *Febrile* seizures are caused by high fevers, tend to run in families and usually occur in children under five years old. If a febrile seizure is generalized (not focal) and lasts less than 5 minutes, it usually is not associated with permanent neurologic dysfunction. *Afebrile* seizures (occurring without a fever) are much more likely to result in residual seizure disorders that are associated with permanent brain injury, especially when they cannot be controlled with medication.

CROHN'S DISEASE - A chronic inflammatory bowel disease characterized by abdominal pain, recurrent diarrhea, fever, loss of appetite, and weight loss. Sometimes arthritis, anemia and growth retardation may occur, especially in children. The cause of Crohn's disease is unknown but it is thought that immunologic, infectious, dietary and genetic predisposition factors may be involved. There is no specific cure or therapy although diet therapy, antibiotics, steroids and surgery have been used. Crohn's disease was only recognized as a separate disease entity several decades ago and is reported to be occurring with increasing frequency in western populations.

DEMYELINATION - The myelin that sheaths many nerve fibers helps the transmission of neural impulses. If the myelin sheath is damaged through traumatic injury, metabolic disorders, toxic insult, viral or bacteria infection or vaccination, it can cause degeneration or *demyelination.* Two well known demyelinating diseases are multiple sclerosis and Guillain-Barre syndrome (See Guillain-Barre syndrome). *Acute disseminated encephalomyelitis* involves demyelination and usually follows a viral infection or vaccination, suggesting an immunologic cause. Symptoms usually begin within days or weeks of vaccination. Sometimes remyelination occurs, with regeneration of the myelin and complete recovery. But often demyelination is irreversible and leads to permanent brain dysfunction or death.

ENCEPHALITIS - Inflammation of the brain which causes swelling in the brain. Tiny hemorrhages can be found scattered throughout the brain, brainstem, cerebellum and sometimes the spinal cord. Encephalitis is thought to usually be caused by a virus; however, a virus is identified as the cause of encephalitis in less than half the cases. There are also noninfectious causes of encephalitis including lead poisoning, brain tumors, multiple sclerosis and vaccine reactions (which are thought to have an immunologic mechanism). Symptoms include alterations in consciousness such as deep sleep alternating with irritability, personality changes, seizures, severe headache, confusion, and partial paralysis. Recovery can be complete without any lasting damage; or varying degrees of permanent brain dysfunction can occur which may include neurologic, behavioral, educational, motor, sensory and self-care dysfunctions. In the most severe cases of encephalitis, the symptoms can progress to stupor, coma and death.

ENCEPHALOMYELITIS - Inflammation of the brain and spinal cord with the same symptoms described in encephalitis above. Destruction or loss of the myelin sheath of a nerve or nerves can be involved with varying degrees of permanent brain dysfunction.

ENCEPHALOPATHY - Any degenerative disease of the brain. Conditions which can lead to encephalopathy include encephalitis, encephalomyelitis, meningitis, convulsions (seizures), head trauma, metabolic disorders, and other illnesses or conditions which cause interference with normal brain function. Sometimes the term encephalopathy is used when brain dysfunction occurs without brain inflammation. Signs of encephalopathy include significant alterations in behavior or consciousness such as prolonged deep sleep alternating with high pitched screaming or hyperactivity and inability to sleep; unconsciousness, stupor, or coma; dramatic personality changes; severe headache; mental confusion; convulsions; partial paralysis and other neurologic signs. Some individuals suffer an acute encephalopathy and are left with few residual effects but many others are left with permanent disabilities including neurologic, behavioral, educational, motor, sensory and self care dysfunctions, including residual seizure disorders.

ERYTHEMA MULTIFORME - An inflammation of the skin or mucous membranes characterized by red circular discolorations of the skin, fluid-filled skin lesions and blisters. Erythema multiforme is associated with infections and drug and vaccine reactions. Symptoms develop suddenly with lesions appearing on the palms of hands and soles of feet and on the face. Itching may occur along with fatigue, joint pain and fever. Attacks can last only a few days or 2 to 4 weeks and may recur. A severe form of erythema multiforme is *Steven-Johnson syndrome*, which involves lesions in the mouth, throat and eyes. The victim may be unable to eat or close the mouth and the eyes may be swollen shut, sometimes resulting in vision loss or, rarely, death.

GUILLAIN-BARRE SYNDROME - Guillain-Barre syndrome (GBS) is a rapidly progressing form of polyneuropathy (see Neuropathy) that can be caused by infections, surgery or vaccination. It is thought to be the most frequently acquired inflammatory demyelinating neuropathy (See Demyelination) and the weight of evidence suggests most cases are immune mediated. Following the 1976-77 national Swine Flu vaccination campaign, there was an increase in the incidence of GBS. At least one influenza vaccine manufacturer warns that persons who have a history of GBS should not be given influenza virus vaccine.

GBS is characterized by muscle weakness, numbness, pain and paralysis. Symptoms may not begin for 1 to 4 weeks following vaccination and then come on suddenly over the course of a day and may continue to progress for several days up to 3 or 4 weeks. Symptoms begin in both legs and may progress up to the arms with signs includ-

74

ing an unsteady gait, burning, prickling and tingling sensations and sometimes paralysis of one or more limbs or of the face. In some cases GBS starts in the arms or cranial nerves and progresses downward to the legs. More than 50 percent of GBS cases involve facial paralysis, sometimes with involvement of the tongue and eye nerves. From 5 to 10 percent of victims require intubation for respiratory failure and occasionally there is temporary bladder paralysis.

Treatment for GBS includes heat to help relieve pain and physical therapy. Recovery lasts several months and can be complete without lasting health problems. It is estimated that 15 to 30 percent of adult victims have some form of chronic weakness at the end of 3 years (the percentage is higher for children). Residual disabilities may require long term physical therapy, orthopedic appliances or corrective surgery. About 10 percent of all victims relapse and enter a chronic state of relapsing polyneuropathy. Less than 5 percent of GBS cases end in death.

HEMOLYTIC ANEMIA - This form of severe anemia is characterized by premature death of the red blood cells and inability of the bone marrow to produce more blood cells quickly enough to replace those that have died. It can be caused by an infection, chemotherapy or occur as part of an autoimmune process. Signs of acute, severe hemolytic anemia can include chills, fever, pain in the back and abdomen, irritability, vomiting, and shock. In reported cases, hemolytic anemia after vaccination occurred within 4 days to three weeks of vaccination.

HERPES ZOSTER - Herpes zoster, also known as shingles, is caused by the varicella zoster virus, the virus which causes chickenpox. For the majority of individuals who recover from chickenpox in childhood, the varicella zoster virus remains inactive in the body throughout life. However, sometimes the varicella zoster virus can be reactivated in adulthood and take the form of herpes zoster (shingles). A very painful skin disorder that causes skin lesions, shingles lasts from 7 to 10 days with recovery taking up to 4 weeks. While most lesions are on the trunk of the body, sometimes lesions may appear on the face, in the mouth, eye or tongue. Severe complications occur most frequently in older adults, including neuralgia and other forms of central nervous system involvement characterized by headache, fever, meningitis and vomiting. Immune compromised individuals, such as those with cancer, are at high risk of complications.

HIGH PITCHED SCREAMING - High pitched screaming is a common but serious reaction to the DPT vaccine which has been reported in the medical literature for more than 50 years. Often Identical to the *cri encephalique* (encephalitic scream) which accompanies some cases of encephalitis in babies and is thought to be an indication of central nervous system irritation, it is characterized by a thin, eerie high pitched wailing cry that is very different from a baby's normal cry. Sometimes babies suffer bouts of high pitched screaming alternating with periods of deep sleep or unconsciousness.

HYPERSENSITIVITY SYNDROME (SERUM-LIKE SICKNESS) - An allergic reaction usually appearing 7 to 12 days after drug therapy or vaccination characterized by fever, joint pain, skin rash and swollen lymph nodes. Hives, swelling and pain in the joints, mild fever for 1 or 2 days, abdominal pain and diarrhea may occur. Complications including peripheral neuritis may cause permanent nerve injury.

HYPOTONIC/HYPORESPONSIVE EPISODES (SHOCK/COLLAPSE) - Hypotonic/hyporesponsive episodes (HHE), which are also described as shock/collapse, are characterized by loss of consciousness accompanied by paleness and limpness of the body. The child may turn bluish and breathing can be very shallow. Fever can be present but often the child's skin is cold. Sometimes after a DPT shot, a child will alternate between HHE and bouts of prolonged crying or high pitched screaming. One U.S. study found that 1 in 1,750 DPT shots is followed by an HHE. Although the biological mechanism for HHE is not known, frequent reports of HHE following DPT vaccination in the medical literature led the Institute of Medicine to conclude in 1991 that DPT vaccine causes HHE. It is not known how many children who suffer HHE go on to exhibit residual neurologic dysfunction.

INSULIN DEPENDENT DIABETES MELLITUS (Juvenile diabetes) - Insulin Dependent Diabetes Mellitus (IDDM), also known as juvenile diabetes or Type 1 diabetes, is a chronic degenerative disease in which the body is unable to produce insulin and cannot properly metabolize blood sugar (glucose). The condition is thought to result from damage to the pancreas caused by an autoimmune reaction in which the insulin producing cells of the pancreas have been destroyed and cannot produce any more insulin. Some scientists have suggested this autoimmunity is triggered by a viral infection or some other kind of insult to the immune system causing it to malfunction. Genetic predisposition may also be involved. Annual incidence of IDDM in the U.S. is about 12 to 14 new cases per 100,000 children up to age 16 years. Symptoms include excessive thirst, hunger, urination and dehydration often with unexplained weight loss. Treatment includes life-long daily injections of insulin. Complications of diabetes can lead to heart and kidney disease, strokes, cataracts, neuropathy, loss of limbs, hearing loss, blindness and death.

LEARNING DISABILITIES - A federal law, used to diagnose learning disabilities in a child for the purpose of funding special education programs, defines learning disabilities as a disorder "in understanding or using language, spoken or written" that may "manifest itself in imperfect ability to listen, think, speak, read, write, spell or do mathematical calculations." Learning disabilities have also been defined as "minimal brain dysfunction" characterized by "certain aberrations of behavior and/or cognitive functioning resulting from milder forms of central nervous system (CNS) dysfunction or developmental deviation." The cause of learning disabilities is the subject of debate among medical doctors but it is thought that a variety of factors are involved including genetic predisposition, biochemical irregularities, perinatal brain insults, viral and bacterial diseases or other insults to the central nervous system during its early development. Learning disabilities, accompanied by attention span deficit, dyslexia, poor memory, clumsiness, sleep disturbances, impulsiveness and emotional lability have all been associated with minimal brain damage in individuals who have had encephalitis, encephalopathy, or other neurologic or immunologic insult occurring during the course of a viral or bacterial infection, exposure to toxins or chemicals or following neurological reactions to vaccinations.

LUPUS - An inflammatory connective tissue disorder that occurs predominately in young women, but also occurs in children. Its precise cause is unknown but lupus is thought to be an autoimmune disorder. The incidence of lupus is increasing around the world and is becoming as common as rheumatoid arthritis. Lupus may occur suddenly after an infection with fever and fatigue or may develop over months or years. Symptoms include fatigue; nausea; weight loss; arthritis; skin and mucus membrane lesions; sensitivity to light; headaches; epilepsy; and lung, heart, kidney and blood disorder problems. There is no cure for lupus and the overall survival rate is about 70 percent after 10 years. Infections and kidney failure are the leading causes of death.

MULTIPLE SCLEROSIS - Multiple sclerosis (MS) is a chronic demyelinating disease which is thought to be immune mediated or caused by an infection but a definitive cause remains unknown. Multiple lesions, old and new, throughout the brain (brainstem, cerebellum, spinal cord) with a systematic breakdown in myelin characterizes MS. A disease that occurs more frequently in women than in men, it usually appears between the ages of 20 and 40. Brain MRI scans are abnormal in more than 90 percent of MS victims, showing brain tissue damage that indicates inflammation has damaged the blood brain barrier.

The first symptom of MS is often an episode of optic neuritis (See Optic Neuritis) with loss of vision in one eye, sometimes accompanied by pain with eye movement. Several weeks, months or years later, more involved symptoms begin including chronic fatigue; sharp pain, weakness, numbness, tingling, burning, itching and involuntary twitching of various parts of the face, hands, and legs; paralysis; loss of vision from one or both eyes or double vision; involuntary rapid movement of the eyeballs; tremors; dizziness, imbalance, incoordination; slurred speech; spasms; bladder and bowel dysfunction; muscle weakness; seizures; personality changes including depression and other neurologic signs. Symptoms may come and go over a period of years with progressive deterioration and disability in 20 to 50 percent of cases after 10 years. About 15 to 25 percent of MS victims have a relatively mild form of the disease. Milder cases may go into remission and have no apparent disability even after 25 years.

NEURITIS - Inflammation of a nerve or noninflammatory lesions of the peripheral nervous system.

NEUROPATHY - Any functional disturbances or pathological changes in the peripheral nervous system characterized by pain, weakness, and numbness causing loss of sensation, muscle weakness and atrophy (wasting/shrinking) and paralysis. There are different kinds of neuropathies, including *mononeuropathy* (involving a single nerve) and *polyneuropathy* (involving many nerves). Recovery is slow and can be complete but some kinds of neuropathy end in permanent disability.

78

OPTIC NEURITIS - This syndrome is characterized by rapid loss of vision over hours or days in one or both eyes caused by demyelination of the optic nerve fibers. Victims complain that everything looks like it is covered with a veil or haze. Sometimes there is pain with eye movement. In a high percentage of patients no cause can be found and many regain full vision within weeks but others are left with partial vision loss. About 15 to 40 percent develop other symptoms consistent with multiple sclerosis within 10 to 15 years.

ORCHITIS - Inflammation of the testes (orchitis) can occur during or following mumps infection, usually 7 to 10 days after onset of mumps. Approximately 20 to 35 percent of males who get mumps after puberty suffer this complication. Headache, nausea, vomiting and high fever can accompany swelling and pain in testicles, which lasts for 3 to 7 days. Recovery is usually complete but, rarely, sterility occurs.

OTITIS MEDIA - Inflammation of the middle ear, otitis media is caused by a bacterial or viral infection that is usually secondary to an upper respiratory infection. Severe earache, high fever, nausea, vomiting and diarrhea are symptoms in young children. Serious complications can include hearing loss, facial paralysis, meningitis, and brain abscess and may be preceded by severe headache, dizziness, sudden hearing loss, chills and high fever.

PERIPHERAL MONONEUROPATHY - Sensory loss, muscle weakness, atrophy (wasting/shrinking) and decreased deep tendon reflexes characterize peripheral nerve disease. Peripheral mononeuropathy involves disease of a single nerve. (See Neuritis, Neuropathy.)

PNEUMONITIS - Also known as pneumonia, pneumonitis is caused by a bacteria or virus that results in a respiratory infection involving the lungs. The most frequent common infection that can result in death, pneumonia symptoms include chest congestion, severe chills, high fever, pain and difficulty breathing, coughing and vomiting up of large amounts of mucous. Antibiotics are usually used to try to control the infection, which can end in death for about 5 percent of patients. Children under one year and adults over 60 years, those with immune disorders or other serious diseases are at increased risk for death from pneumonia.

RADICULONEURITIS - Acute febrile (with fever) polyneuritis (inflammation of many nerves simultaneously).

RESIDUAL SEIZURE DISORDER - See *CONVULSIONS (SEIZURES)*

RETINITIS - Inflammation of the retina, the innermost tunic of the eyeball containing the neural elements for reception and transmission of visual stimuli.

REYE'S SYNDROME - Reye's syndrome was first identified and described as a separate pathologic entity in 1963. It is characterized by an acute encephalopathy and dysfunction of the liver that can follow some acute viral infections. Although its cause is unknown, it is associated with viral infections (chicken pox, influenza, Epstein-Barr virus), toxins, salicylates (such as aspirin), and metabolic defects. Commonly Reye's begins around day 6 of an upper respiratory infection with severe nausea and vomiting and sudden change in mental functioning with signs including disorientation, agitation, amnesia, extreme lethargy (sleepiness) which can progress to unresponsiveness, coma, and, sometimes, death. Because Reye's syndrome is most common in children under 18 years, it is recommended that aspirin never be given to children who are sick with viral infections.

SENSORINEURAL DEAFNESS - Hearing loss due to a lesion in the inner ear or the 8th nerve. Hearing loss ranges from mild to moderate to severe.

SPINAL TAP (LUMBAR PUNCTURE) - This diagnostic medical procedure involves using a needle to puncture the lumbar region of the spinal cord and withdraw cerebral spinal fluid (CSF) for evaluation to determine if the individual has a viral or bacterial infection in the brain. A sometimes risky and often very painful procedure when no anesthetic is used, it is often only performed after a CT scan (computed tomographic x-ray) or MRI (magnetic resonance imaging) of the brain has been taken to rule out any brain conditions, such as high CSF pressure caused by a tumor or other problems, which could make a spinal tap very dangerous.

SUBACUTE SCLEROSING PANENCEPHALITIS - This is a rare, progressive and ultimately fatal disease of children and adolescents that has long been suspected of being caused by viral infection. Atypical measles virus or a virus closely related to measles virus has been recovered from the brains of patients with this disease and scientists say they cannot determine in any given case if the virus is linked to measles disease or live measles vaccination. Subacute sclerosing panencephalitis (SSPE) is considered to be a slow form of measles encephalitis and there can be a delay of up to 1 year or more between the time a person comes into contact with the measles virus before symptoms of SSPE appear. Lesions are found in the gray and white brain matter.

SSPE most often occurs in individuals between the ages of 4 and 20, with 80 percent under age 11. It affects boys 3 to 10 times as often as girls. Symptoms begin gradually with a decline in schoolwork, personality changes, clumsiness and uncoordinated movements, jerking (seizure activity) and vision problems. The individual becomes bedridden within 6 to 9 months and becomes spastic, blind and unable to swallow. Coma follows with death usually caused by lung, urinary tract or other infections. The course of SSPE can last from weeks to years, with the average victim dying within two years. Rarely, a person can remain in a chronic vegetative state for 10 or more years.

SUDDEN INFANT DEATH SYNDROME (SIDS) - The sudden death of an apparently healthy infant or young child which is unexpected and in which an autopsy fails to demonstrate an adequate cause for death. SIDS, also known as "crib death," is the most common diagnosis listed as the cause of death in babies between the ages of 2 weeks and 1 year of age, accounting for 30 percent of all deaths in this age group. Peak incidence of SIDS occurs between two and four months of age. Almost all deaths occur when the infant is sleeping. Although only a small percentage of SIDS victims have a known history of apnea, there is some speculation that a special kind of sleep apnea with irregular heartbeats may be accentuated by poor coordination of the respiratory muscles due to the immaturity of the nervous system. The precise cause of SIDS remains unknown.

THROMBOCYTOPENIA PURPURA - A reduced number of platelets circulating in the blood producing purpura, blotchy red patches on the body caused by the thinned blood seeping into the tissues beneath the skin. Thrombocytopenia purpura can occur following viral infections,or reactions to drugs or vaccines, as part of an autoimmune response. It is most common in children and 60 percent recover within 4 to 6 weeks and more than 90 percent recover in 3 to 6 months. However, severe thrombocytopenia can end in death.

TINNITUS - Perception of sound in the absence of real sound. Often perceived as a buzzing, ringing, roaring, whistling or hissing sound in the ear and hearing loss usually is present. It may occur during infection, drug treatment, head trauma, and certain disease processes.

TRANSVERSE MYELITIS -This is a clinical syndrome characterized by a sudden onset of signs of spinal cord disease and involves demyelination of the spinal cord. It can be associated with multiple sclerosis or acute disseminated encephalomyelitis (see Demyelination). Transverse myelitis has been associated with viral infection, IV drug use and vaccination, but no definitive cause has been found. Symptoms begin with sudden local back pain followed over several days by pain and weakness starting in the feet and moving upward. Bladder and bowel dysfunction and partial paralysis often follow. There is no treatment and many victims are left with significant disabilities.

URTICARIA - Also known as hives, urticaria is essentially anaphylaxis limited to the skin and can be caused by allergies to drugs, insect stings or bites; foods; viral infections; and vaccinations. Symptoms usually begin within minutes or hours of exposure and usually subside within 1 to 7 days. Swelling may occur. If the mucus membranes of the throat are involved, it can be life threatening and immediate treatment with antihistamine and other measures are necessary.

BIBLIOGRAPHY

The following list of references is a partial list of information sources used to compile this booklet. Readers who would like to independently research vaccines and diseases are encouraged to consult a medical library at a college. NVIC also offers books, videos and information packets on specific subjects which may be of interest.

Albonico H, Klein P, Grob Ch, Pewsner D. 1992. The Immunisation Campaign against Measles, Mumps and Rubella, Coercion leading to Uncertainty: Medical Objections to a Continued MMR Immunisation Campaign in Switzerland. *Journal of Anthroposophic Medicine* 9(1) Spring.

Alderslade R, Bellman MH, Rawson NSB, Ross EM, Miller DL. 1981. *The National Childhood Encephalopathy Study*: a report on 1000 cases of serious neurological disorders in infants and young children from the NCES research team. In: Whooping Cough: Reports from the Committee on the Safety of Medicines and the Joint Committee on Vaccination and Immunisation. Department of Health and Social Security. London: Her Majesty's Stationery Office.

American Academy of Pediatrics. 1994. *The Red Book*. Report of the Committee on Infectious Diseases, 23rd edition. Peter G, ed. Elk Grove, IL: American Academy of Pediatrics.

Baraff LJ, Cherry JD. 1979. Nature and rates of adverse reactions associated with pertussis immunization. In: Manclark CR and Hill JC, eds. International Symposium on Pertussis. US Department of Health, Education and Welfare Publication No. (NIH) 79-1830. Washington, DC: US Government Printing Office.

Berkow R, ed. 1987. Pertussis. *Merck Manual of Diagnosis and Therapy*, 15th edition. Rahway, NJ: Merck Sharpe & Dohme Research Laboratories.

Braunwald E, Isselbacher KJ, Petersdorf RG, Wilson JD, Martin JB, Fauci AS, eds. 1987. *Harrison's Principles of Internal Medicine*. New York: McGraw-Hill, Inc.

Burton Goldberg Group, ed. 1994. *Alternative Medicine: The Definitive Guide.* Puyallup: Future Medicine Publishing, Inc.

Carbone M, Rizzo P, Procopia A, et al. 1996. SV-40-like sequences in human bone tumors. *Oncogene*, 12.

Centers for Disease Control. 1987. Pertussis immunization: family history of convulsions and use of antipyretics - supplementary ACIP statement. *Morbidity and Mortality Weekly Report* 36.

Centers or Disease Control. 1992. Pertussis Vaccination: Acellular Pertussis Vaccine for Reinforcing and Booster Use - Supplementary ACIP Statement. *Morbidity and Mortality Weekly Report 41* (February 7, 1992).

Centers for Disease Control. 1995. Recommended Childhood Immunization Schedule - United States, 1995. *Morbidity and Mortality Weekly Report* 44 (June 16).

Centers for Disease Control. 1995. Summary of Notifiable Diseases, United States - 1994. *Morbidity and Mortality Weekly Report* 43 (October 6).

Centers for Disease Control. 1996. Measles - United States, 1995. *Morbidity and Mortality Weekly Report* 45 (April 19).

Centers for Disease Control. 1996. Prevention of Varicella - Recommendations of the Advisory Committee on Immunization Practices (ACIP). *Morbidity and Mortality Weekly Report* 45 (July 12).

Centers for Disease Control. 1996. Update: Vaccine Side Effects, Adverse Reactions, Contraindications, and Precautions - Recommendations of the Advisory Committee on Immunization Practices (ACIP). *Morbidity and Mortality Weekly Report* 45 (September 6).

Centers for Disease Control. 1996. Summary of Notifiable Diseases, United States - 1995. *Morbidity and Mortality Weekly Report 44* (October 25).

Centers for Disease Control. 1996. Progress Toward Elimination of Haemophilus influenzae Type b Disease Among Infants and Children - United States, 1987-1995. *Morbidity and Mortality Weekly Report* 45 (October 25).

Clements SD and Peters JE. 1981. Syndromes of minimal brain dysfunction. In *Brain dysfunction in children: Etiology, diagnosis, and management.* New York: Raven Press.

Cody CL, Baraff LJ, Cherry JD, Marcy SM, Manclark CR. 1981. Nature and rates of adverse reactions associated with DTP and DT immunizations in infants and children. *Pediatrics* 68:650-660.

Connaught Laboratories, Inc. Diphtheria and tetanus toxoids and pertussis vaccine adsorbed USP (*Package Insert* July 1986).

Connaught Laboratories, Inc. Polio Virus Vaccine Inactivated: IPOL (*Package Insert* December 1990).

Connaught Laboratories, Inc. Diphtheria and tetanus toxoids and acellular pertussis vaccine adsorbed: TRIPEDIA (*Package Insert* July 1996).

Coulter HL & Fisher BL. 1985. *DPT: A Shot in the Dark.* San Diego: Harcourt Brace Jovanovich.

DeGowin RL. 1987. *DeGowin & DeGowin's Diagnostic Examination.* New York: Macmillan Publishing Company.

Fisher BL, ed. 1996. Microbiologist Issues a Challenge to Science: Did the First Oral Polio Vaccine Lots Contaminated with Monkey Viruses Create a Monkey-Human Hybrid Called HIV-1? *THE VACCINE REACTION,* National Vaccine Information Center (April).

Herroelen L, DeKeyser J, Ebinger G. 1991. Central-nervous system demyelination after immunisation with recombinant hepatitis B vaccine. *The Lancet* 338 (November 9): 1174-1175.

Institute of Medicine. 1991. *Adverse Effects of Pertussis and Rubella Vaccines.* Washington, DC: National Academy Press.

Institute of Medicine. 1994. *Adverse Effects Associated with Childhood Vaccines: Evidence Bearing on Causality.* Washington, D.C: National Academy Press.

Institute of Medicine. 1994. *DPT Vaccine and Chronic Nervous System Dysfunction: A New Analysis.* Washington, D.C.: National Academy Press.

Institute of Medicine. 1996. *Options for Poliomyelitis Vaccination in the United States.* Washington, D.C.: National Academy Press.

Johnson H. 1996. *Osler's Web: Inside the Labyrinth of the Chronic Fatigue Syndrome Epidemic.* New York: Crown Publishers, Inc.

Kyle W. 1992. Simian retroviruses, poliovaccine, and origin of AIDS. *The Lancet* 339:March 7.

Lederle Laboratories Division, American Cyanamid Co. Poliovirus Vaccine Live Oral Trivalent: ORIMUNE (*Package Insert* October 1992).

Lederle Laboratories Division, American Cyanamid Co. Diphtheria and Tetanus Toxoids Adsorbed Purogenated (*Package Insert* May 1988).

Lederle Laboratories Division, American Cyanamid Co. Diphtheria and Tetanus Toxoids and Pertussis Vaccine Adsorbed: TRI-IMMUNOL (*Package Insert* August 1991).

Lederle Laboratories Division, American Cyanamid Co. Diphtheria and Tetanus Toxoids and Acellular Pertussis Vaccine Adsorbed: ACEL-IMUNE (*Package Insert* January 1992).

Lederle-Praxis Biologicals, Inc., Division of American Cyanamid Co. Haemophilus b Conjugate Vaccine: HibTITER (*Package Insert* April 1994).

Martin WJ, Ahmed KN, Zeng LC, et al. 1995. African green monkey origin of the atypical cytopathic 'stealth virus' isolated from a patient with chronic fatigue syndrome. *Clinical Diagnostic Virology* 4: 93-103.

Medical Economics Data. 1994. *Physicians' Desk Reference.* Montvale: Medical Economics Data Production Co.

Menkes JH, Kinsbourne M. 1990. Workshop on neurologic complications of pertussis and pertussis vaccination. *Neuropediatrics* 21: 171-176.

Merck & Co., Inc. Measles, Mumps and Rubella Virus Vaccine Live, MSD: ATTENUVAX, MUMPSVAX, MERUVAX (*Product Insert* March 1991).

Merck & Co., Inc. Hepatitis B Vaccine (Recombinant): RECOMBIVAX HB (*Package Insert* March 1993).

86

Merck & Co., Inc. Varicella Virus Vaccine Live (Oka/Merck): VARIVAX (*Package Insert* March 1995).

Merck Research Laboratories. 1987. *The Merck Manual.* Rahway: Merck & Co.

Miller DL, Ross EM, Alderslade R, Bellman MH, Rawson HSB. 1981. Pertussis immunisation and serious acute neurological illness in children. *British Medical Journal* 282: 1595-1599.

Montinari M, Favoino B, Roberto A. 1996. Diagnostic Role of Immunogenetics in Post-Vaccine Diseases of the Central Nervous System (CNS): Preliminary Results. *Mediterranean Journal of Surgery and Medicine* 2: 69-72.

Mothering Magazine. *1996. Vaccination: The Issue of Our Times* (Summer).

United States Department of Health and Human Services, National Institute of Allergy and Infectious Diseases, National Institutes of Health Pertussis Conference. Acellular Pertussis Vaccine Trials: Results and Impact on U.S. Public Health, June 3-5, 1996.

Riskind P. 1996. Multiple Sclerosis: The Immure System's Terrible Mistake. *ON THE BRAIN,* Harvard Mahoney Neuroscience Institute (Fall).

Rock A. 1996. The Lethal Dangers of the Billion Dollar Vaccine Business. *Money Magazine* (December).

Shorter E. 1987. *The Health Century.* New York: Doubleday.

Thompson NP, Montgomery SM, Pounder RE, Wakefield AJ. 1995. Is measles vaccination a risk factor for inflammatory bowel disease? *The Lancet* 345 (April 29): 1071-1074.

Tishon A, Manchester M, Scheiflinger F, Oldston M. 1996. A model of measles virus-induced immunosuppression: Enhanced susceptibility of neonatal human PBLs. *Nature Medicine* 2 (11): 1250-1254.

Torch WC. 1982. Diphtheria-pertussis-tetanus (DPT) immunization: A potential cause of the sudden infant death syndrome (SIDS). American Academy of Neurology, 34th Annual Meeting, April 25-May 1. *Neurology* 32(4): pt.2.

Trollfors B. 1984. Bordetella pertussis whole cell vaccines: efficacy and toxicity. *Acta Paediatrica Scandinavia* 73:417-425.

Wechsler P. 1996. Shot in the Dark. *New York Magazine* (November 11).

Wyeth Laboratories, Inc. Influenza Virus Vaccine Trivalent, Types A and B: FLUSHIELD 1996-97 (*Package Insert* May 1996)

About The Author

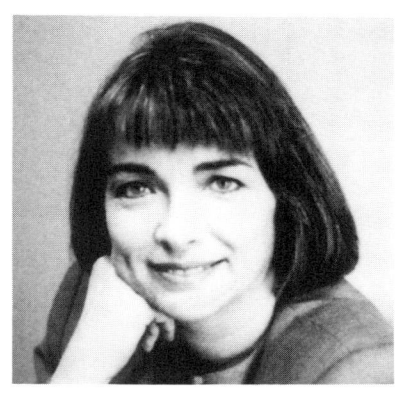

Barbara Loe Fisher is a co-founder and president of the National Vaccine Information Center. She is co-author of <u>DPT: A Shot in the Dark</u> (Harcourt Brace Jovanovich, 1985; Warner, 1986; Avery 1991) and is editor of NVIC's national, bi-monthly newsletter *THE VACCINE REACTION*. During the early 1980's, she helped launch a grassroots movement to bring the issue of vaccine safety to public attention, including leading demonstrations at the Centers for Disease Control in Atlanta and the White House in 1986. Later that year, Congress passed the National Childhood Vaccine Injury Act of 1986.

She served on the National Vaccine Advisory Committee for four years; was appointed to the Institute of Medicine Vaccine Safety Forum in 1995; and has represented health care consumers concerned about vaccine safety at many scientific conferences, government meetings and legislative hearings. She has appeared on radio and television programs speaking about vaccine safety, including the "Today Show," CBS Evening News, "Nightline," and "Regis Philbin" and has contributed to numerous newspaper and magazine articles providing vaccine information to the public. She is an active public speaker at health care conferences and town meetings, defending the human right of citizens to make informed, independent health care choices for themselves and their children, including the right to informed consent to vaccination.

Barbara is the mother of three children. Her oldest son was left with multiple learning disabilities and attention deficit disorder after a severe reaction to his fourth DPT shot in 1980 when he was two and a half years old.

-cut here-

NATIONAL VACCINE INFORMATION CENTER

512 W. Maple Avenue, #206, Vienna, VA 22180

800-909-SHOT   www.909shot.com

☐ Yes, I want to become a NEW member of NVIC to help prevent vaccine injuries and death through public education, defend the right to informed consent to vaccination and get *THE VACCINE REACTION* newsletter.

☐ $25 Individual
To help educate
parents

☐ $50 Professional
To help prevent vaccine
reactions & injuries

☐ $100 Associate
To help obtain the right
to informed consent

☐ $200 Sponsor
To help fund scientific
research

☐ Please send me a copy of **THE CONSUMER'S GUIDE TO CHILDHOOD VACCINES** ($11)

TOTAL ENCLOSED: $_____

NAME _____ DATE: _____

ADDRESS: _____

CITY: _____ STATE: _____ ZIP: _____ TELEPHONE:(____) _____

CREDIT CARD NUMBER: _____ EXP. DATE: _____

Make checks payable to NVIC. Add $10 for all orders outside USA. U. S. Funds only.
Return to: The National Vaccine Information Center, 512 W. Maple Ave., Suite 206, Vienna. VA 22180

-cut here-

THE CONSUMER'S GUIDE TO CHILDHOOD VACCINES ORDER FORM

☐ $9.00 per copy (Plus $2.00 shipping) _____ # of copies _____ Total

☐ 10 to 99 copies at $7.50 each _____ # of copies _____ Total

☐ 100-500 copies at $5.50 each _____ # of copies _____ Total

☐ Check   ☐ MC   ☐ VISA   Exp. Date _____ / _____

CARD #: _____

NAME: _____ TEL #: _____

ADDRESS: _____

CITY: _____ STATE: _____ ZIP: _____

Make checks payable to NVIC. Add $5 for all orders outside the USA. U.S Funds only, must be imprinted by your bank.

Return to: The National Vaccine Information Center, 512 West Maple Avenue, #206,

Vienna,VA 22180.   (703) 938-5768 Fax   (703) 938-DPT3

Phone orders: 800-909-SHOT   http://www.909shot.com